American Medical Association

Physicians dedicated to the health of America

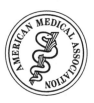

Automating the Medical Record

D1479728

Project Manager/Editor: .... Kay Stanley
Author: .... Tom Landholt, M.D.
Art Director: .... Jeff Weir

Published by:

Coker Publishing, LLC —
in affiliation with The Coker Group
3150 Holcomb Bridge Road, Suite 310
Norcross, Georgia 30071
(770) 242-0118

PUBLISHING
COMPANY

ISBN 0-89970-909-5

American Medical Association Preface

This book and others in the PRACTICE SUCCESS!© Series are designed to offer you concrete, practical information on topics that you may sometimes consider the least important aspect of the profession of medicine—the business of running a medical practice. And in some ways, that's how it should be. The long, hard years you dedicated to medical school and residency training were meant to make you an excellent physician, not an excellent businessperson. Caring for patients is, and always will be, your first priority. Nevertheless, you cannot successfully run a medical practice without planning and without consideration of important business issues. While it takes a minimum of ten years for a person to become a physician, the day a practice opens is the day a physician becomes a small businessperson.

While your many years of superb education probably did not include classes in medical office operations, personnel management, accounting, or business law, these business issues are more important than ever before because the practice of medicine in today's rapidly changing environment is far more complex than ever before. Good business management today is essential to a good medical practice. The physician who ignores basic business principles in operating his or her practice may soon face difficulties with suppliers, employees, the government, or even patients.

Other pressures today force physicians to search for more efficient ways of running their practices. Most physicians find demands on their time increasing tremendously. There is a daily struggle to build a practice that will earn a steady income, to schedule regular working hours, to deliver quality care to patients, and to still have time for relaxation and family.

Developing an efficient practice that runs smoothly makes all these goals attainable. The application of good business planning will enable you to spend more time on those things that are most important to you.

This book and the others in the PRACTICE SUCCESS!© Series are guides to medical practice management for both the new physician and the established physician who wants to improve his or her practice. These books will not provide solutions to every problem that may arise in day-to-day practice. Our goal is to acquaint you with essential business principles and tools, as well as with some new approaches to managing your practice. The knowledge you acquire from this series can be supplemented with information you gather from your colleagues and advisors. You will then be in a position to explore those ideas that promise to achieve the best results for your particular practice situation.

By providing the information in this book and others, the American Medical Association (AMA) is not endorsing any specific management philosophy or method of delivering health care services. No one approach will meet the objectives of all physicians. Physicians and their staffs should decide for themselves what is the best way to manage their individual practices. Finally, this book does not enunciate AMA policy. The annual Policy Compendium of the AMA sets forth our positions on such issues as contracting, medical ethics, managed care, and practice management.

We hope that this publication will be useful to you.

The American Medical Association

About The Coker Group

THE COKER GROUP is a national provider of health care consultative and management services assisting physicians, hospitals, and health care systems to better position themselves to be successful in a rapidly changing health care environment. THE COKER GROUP offers the following services for its clients:

Programs and Services:

- Physician Network Development

- Practice Appraisals and Valuations

- Acquisition Negotiations

- Physician Employment and Compensation and Contract Design

- Group Practice Development

- Practice Management Services

- Management Services Organization Development; Network Assessments

- Practice Brokering

- Practice Start-ups

- Educational Programs, Seminars, and Workshops

- Health System Medical Staff Development and Manpower Plans

- *PRACTICE SUCCESS!*© and *PRACTICE SUCCESS!*© Series

For more information, contact:

THE
Coker
G R O U P
National Consultants to Healthcare Providers

The Coker Group / 3150 Holcomb Bridge Road / Suite 310
Norcross, Georgia 30071 / (800) 345-5829

http://www.cokergroup.com

About the Book _____

Automating the Medical Record addresses one of the most stimulating topics under discussion in medical practice today: electronic medical records. The underlying issue is not whether computers should be used in medicine. Indeed, computer technology exists in virtually every area of medicine. Rather, the issue is making the transition to a new method of documenting patient care and viewing patient data.

What are physicians' basic underlying concerns?

- We have never done it this way before. Changing routines is difficult and disruptive.

- What happens if I make the wrong product decision? The financial commitment is significant. Investing in a weak or unreliable program is risky.

- Maybe I should wait for additional technological advances. The prudent physician wants to know when is the right time to buy.

- What about my responsibilities to my patients for confidentiality and security? The integrity of the patient-physician relationship is of paramount importance.

In *Automating the Medical Record,* we have established the following goals:

- To lay a foundation for a means of documenting patient care electronically

- To inform the reader of the myriad options and computer components

- To address confidentiality and security issues

This material is an overview of the selection process. We have set successive steps for assessing the benefits of electronic medical records (EMR) and evaluating the currently available software.

Who should read this book?

This publication is for anyone interested or involved in the management of a medical practice. It is a guide to the fundamentals of electronic medical records. Some readers may have no knowledge of computers, while others may be familiar with some aspects of office automation. Typically, the office staff has a greater knowledge of office automation than the physician. This book also lays the groundwork for purchasing the necessary computer hardware and software to operate the practice in an electronic environment. Among those who should read it are the following:

- Practicing physicians

- Owners of medical practices and clinics

- Practice administrators and business managers

- Hospital system practice administrators

Anyone whose interest centers on the "how to" along with the "why"of EMR will benefit greatly from reading this material.

What information can the reader find?

Written from a practicing physician's perspective, this book offers sensible and specific guidance about:

- The reasons to purchase an EMR system
- The requirements for making a transition from the paper chart to the computerized chart
- The steps for evaluating a vendor
- The process of preparing the practice for automation

Is the information current?

Computer technology changes at an amazingly rapid rate—perhaps at a greater rate than in any other industry. However, today's consumer can purchase only what is currently for sale, regardless of what the industry is in the process of developing. This publication examines the hardware and software available to the medical practice today, along with its current applications.

A member of the advisory board of a software company, the author's product review and software development experience make him uniquely aware of what is available currently and what the marketplace will soon offer. He presents an unbiased review of the decision-making process and the technology rather than offering product-specific information.

The *PRACTICE SUCCESS!* Series

This book is a part of a series based on the practice management program titled *PRACTICE SUCCESS!* As publishers, we are committed to providing physicians in medical practice with the most current information concerning topics of interest for the business side of medicine. For more detail on this and other resources available through The Coker Group, contact us at the following address:

The Coker Group, LLC
3150 Holcomb Bridge Road
Suite 310
Norcross, GA 30071
(770) 242-0118

Also, visit our home page on the World Wide Web on the Internet:

http://www.cokergroup.com

Kay Stanley
Editor

About the Author _____

Thomas F. Landholt, M.D., a family practitioner with Steeplechase Family Physicians (an affiliate of Cox Health Systems in Springfield, Missouri) is a nationally recognized author and speaker on electronic medical records and the delivery of patient-focused care. Dr. Landholt's credentials include a baccalaureate degree from St. Louis University and an M.D. from the University of Missouri, Columbia. He completed his residency at Cox Family Practice in Springfield in 1991 and attained his Board Certification in Family Practice the same year.

Dr. Landholt's research, publications, and presentations include: research on "After-hours Phone Calls," presented at the NAPCRG meeting in Quebec City, Quebec, 1990; participation in a national study on ibuprofen, published in the *Journal of the American Medical Association (JAMA)*, 1995; First Author, Clinical Therapeutics, 1994, "A Pharmacoeconomic Comparison of Amoxicillin/ Clavulanate and Cefpodoxime Proxetil in the Treatment of Acute Otitis Media"; and participation in a study on new diabetic oral medication.

I first met Dr. Landholt in 1996 in Nashville, Tennessee, where he was presenting a program to the Medical Group Management Association titled "Perspectives on EMR." His practical approach to complex information captivated his audience of physicians, practice executives, and professional administrators. He put his listeners at ease with his encouraging delivery style and interesting applications.

Dr. Landholt views medical practice as a service industry and patients as consumers. Patients seek medical care because they have needs; they are ill, or injured, or they need preventive care. As consumers, patients want their doctor and his or her staff to treat them well and to respect their time.

Like you, Dr. Landholt is a physician who works in a busy medical practice. He practices medicine using electronic tools. I think you will appreciate Dr. Landholt's approach to *Automating the Medical Record*. His expertise in the benefits of EMR and his straightforward advice on selecting an information system will serve as a practical resource for the specific needs of your practice.

Kay Stanley
Editor

Overview

What is an *automated medical practice*? What is a computerized medical record? How does the practice that has already invested heavily in management software, with scheduling and billing capabilities (and more), decide to take the next step in automation—electronic medical records? What will happen to the thousands of paper charts that have always been the center of patient care? How will you know the time is right to move forward in the automation of your practice?

Many physicians perceive electronic medical record keeping (EMR) as no more than a computerized version of a paper chart, or believe that the computer record will (or should) look like the paper chart. Nothing, however, could be further from the truth. More than just the "next step" in medical records management, EMR can transform the way physicians practice.

And yet, some physicians, comfortable only with seeing and doing things the same old way, are initially disturbed by having to use information in a new "landscape."

Sometimes the office staff, out of resistance to change, can be the biggest barrier to successful EMR implementation. This is especially true for long-term employees who are comfortable with familiar procedures and routines. (Ironically, once the electronic medical records system is in place, the staff often becomes its greatest proponent because of the benefits it brings to the practice.)

On the other hand, your office staff may already be "leaps and bounds" ahead of you in their knowledge of and interest in office automation. They may already be aware of the time savings and benefits computerized patient charts will bring to practice operations. They may be anxiously awaiting the time when you are ready to move forward into the EMR environment.

Understanding a computerized record requires a philosophical change in the way the physician collects, manages, and views patient data. During the first six months after start-up, the changes may feel awkward and alien. In fact, however, the new methods are superior because they allow the physician to use the patient data more effectively. In the end, both physician and patient benefit from the conversion to EMR.

So long as other practices send paper charts and paper lab reports to your practice, you will have paper to handle. However, you can substantially reduce the amount of paper in your practice, the time it takes to handle it, and the room it takes to store it by converting to the electronic mode. As more practices computerize and more physicians venture into the world of electronic records, your opportunities to share information electronically will increase. The electronic market is growing at a rate of 70 percent annually, and the time is coming when paper will no longer be the accepted conduit for transferring patient information. In the future, patient information will be accessible through system interfaces and will reflect the continuum of patient care.

> *"Resistance is futile."*
> — Star Trek

A *successful* transition from paper charts to electronic medical records is founded on these guidelines:

1. Start with a plan.

2. Set objectives.

3. Follow a disciplined evaluation process.

4. When using multiple vendors, select vendors with similar cultures and attitudes.

5. Develop a plan for your employees and your long-term staffing requirements.

6. Define the scope of the tasks to be considered and the future areas that you may include.

7. Use the "partnership" concept to create a mutually beneficial environment with your vendor.

8. Insist on service agreements; maintain a well-trained staff to keep your system up and running.

9. Develop a plan for application. Recognize that communications will be a critical success factor.

10. Plan for change.

Practice advantages will come from the use and application of technology. Don't be left behind. A few months after you automate your medical practice, you will ask yourself, "How did I ever function without it?"

Table of Contents

CHAPTER 1

Building Support for Electronic Medical Records

Electronic Patient Encounters

Electronic patient encounters are not things of the future; they are here now. However, if the concept of an electronic medical record is unfamiliar to you, you may have difficulty envisioning the experience. Moving from paper to computer requires a shift in thinking and a revolution in the traditional way that a practice handles its patients. A typical electronic encounter in your office might occur in the following way:

Mrs. Jones, whose husband is your patient, calls to make a "new patient" appointment for herself. As the receptionist speaks with Mrs. Jones, she schedules the office visit and creates an electronic medical record for Mrs. Jones. Personal information, such as address, telephone numbers, and background data necessary for patient population studies come directly from Mr. Jones's chart, as the computer electronically links the two as a family.

When Mrs. Jones arrives for her appointment, she enters a relaxed and friendly office environment where she observes that the receptionist greets other patients in the waiting area by name. Soon afterward, the front office personnel photograph Mrs. Jones. Later, when she sees her photograph on the computer monitor as part of her chart, she understands how the staff recognizes arriving patients.

The receptionist clicks on the screen to document the time Mrs. Jones checks in for her appointment. This action automatically notifies the nurse that Mrs. Jones is waiting in the reception area.

After the nurse escorts Mrs. Jones to the examining room, she takes vital signs and enters them directly into the computer terminal. The nurse then questions Mrs. Jones about her allergies, current medications, and medical history and adds this information to her electronic "chart."

When the physician enters the exam room, the encounter begins with a review of the medical chart summary. This happens quite quickly, since he has already reviewed the new information the nurse placed in the chart from the terminal in his office. The doctor asks Mrs. Jones a few additional questions while they look together at her medical history on the computer terminal in the exam room.

Then the physician examines Mrs. Jones and, using templates on the terminal, enters all of the history and physical findings into the chart with a point and click of the mouse. He prescribes medication for her by choosing from a database accessed through the computer program. The EMR program warns him of a potential drug-drug interaction and prints a handout of precautions for the patient. As the physician selects and enters the appropriate diagnosis code(s), he automatically prints a patient handout about Mrs. Jones's condition.

On the way out of the office, the front office staff tell Mrs. Jones that they have transmitted her prescriptions to her pharmacy, which should have them ready when she gets there. They also give her an updated patient identification card with all of her current medical information to place into her wallet. Seeing the diagnosis "pharyngitis" update on her screen, the receptionist bids Mrs. Jones farewell, saying she hopes that her throat improves quickly.

By this time, the staff has already electronically submitted all of the International Classifications of Diseases, 9th Revision, Clinical Modification (ICD-9-CM) and Current Procedural Terminology (CPT™) codes for her visit to her insurance carrier. Within 48 hours of her appointment, the payer will post the payment back to the office account. Mrs. Jones's medical record is completely current by the time she leaves the physician's office. At the end of the day, diagnoses, medications, side effects, blood pressure, and other patient information from the EMR are deposited into a central database.

The health care plan with which Mrs. Jones is enrolled is vitally interested in the medication that she takes for her condition. The plan is aware of a newly released medication and wants to evaluate whether it is a better alternative for her. To begin the process, the health care system queries the database for certain kinds of information. Using the data collected, the health care system, over a matter of months, determines through comparison studies that the older medication is far more effective for Mrs. Jones's condition and, through its "intranet," generates a bulletin to all providers reporting the efficacy of the medication.

The following week, Mrs. Jones sees a program on television that tells about the new medication. Wondering why her doctor is not treating her with the medication, she calls her physician to ask about this new "wonder drug." With the information bulletin on her screen, the nurse is able to provide Mrs. Jones with facts from the data collected and reassures her that the physician has considered all the alternative medications and prescribed in her best interest. As a result, Mrs. Jones is a happy, satisfied patient.

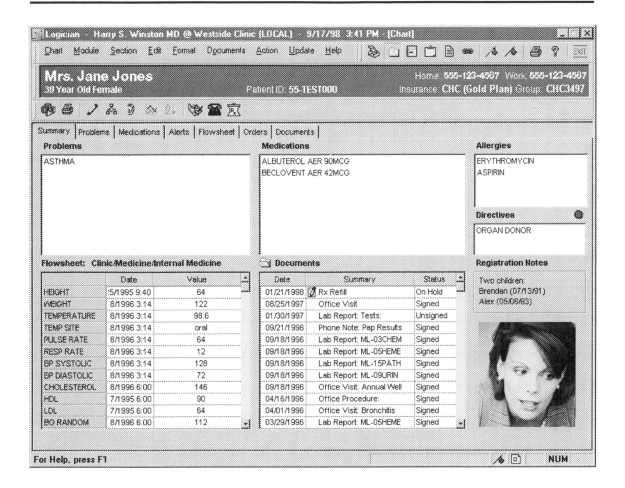

The medical profession requires that doctors have ready access to a host of data and maintain access to them over time. The medical record as a paper chart, until recently the center of patient care, has never been a perfect tool for handling the myriad graphic and data elements inherent to medicine. In reality, physicians rely on the paper chart for a function it cannot aptly serve due to its physical limitations.

With electronic medical office software now available and functional, the "electronic revolution" is sweeping medicine quickly, transforming the practice environment. At last it is possible to set up a system that will improve the quality of data and access to them, increase efficiency, and save time.

As one part of the information systems package, the electronic medical record (EMR), or the computerized patient record (CPR) as it is often referred to, *will be* the cornerstone of office automation. Ease of use — having simple access to information and to individuals who can provide support when necessary — is the key factor for smoothly moving from the paper chart to the "paperless chart." Anticipating and planning ensure that a transition to EMR will be calm and productive.

In the remainder of this chapter, we will address gaining support for EMR, first from physicians, then from the practice staff. Using practical applications, we will explain various uses for EMR and the benefits your practice will derive from its features.

Keys to Acceptance

Some physicians and staff may initially resist computerization, especially when the perception is that a change requires additional investment in time and transition from comfortable routines. A successful move from paper to computerization begins with understanding of the dynamics involved in that transition.

Mark Leavitt, M.D., Ph.D., writes that there are three keys to physician and staff acceptance of the use of the electronic medical record.

Key 1: The rational factors

Benefits:

- Improved access to the record

- Legibility and organization of data

- Availability of decision support

- Connectivity with other providers

- Increased productivity

- Decreased labor needs

- Improved customer service

- Availability of quality and outcomes data

Obstacles:

- Cost of the hardware, software, and network infrastructure

- Time needed for training

- Lost productivity during conversion

Based on these benefits and obstacles, one can create a return-on-investment analysis that shows the rational value of changing to electronic records — the first key to acceptance. However, experience shows that a positive return on investment alone is not sufficient reason for a "go" decision, nor does it guarantee successful implementation and use of EMR. Emotional and inertial factors must also be considered.

Key 2: The emotional factor

The move from paper-based records to EMR is a drastic change and touches directly on what clinicians and staff do.

- Physicians may worry that the computer will dilute their authority and control.

- Physicians may worry that computers will collect data that payers and administrators can use to gain control over them.

- Staff members may fear layoffs as use of computers reduces the number of personnel needed to manage records.

- Physicians and staff who are not computer literate may be concerned about learning to use the system efficiently and whether they might lose status to those more skilled with computers.

Overcoming these barriers requires unmasking people's hidden concerns and addressing them. Often, concern arises from lack of information, and a full explanation of the benefits of automation is all that is needed to help staff understand the benefits of implementing an EMR system. When EMR allows you to reengineer office workflow, for instance, their new speed and efficiency allow staff members more time during the day to cross-train into other areas, to gain new skills with the computer, and to grow professionally into more meaningful roles. Using ROI analysis and incremental steps toward change, you will be able to do much to ease staff uncertainty.

Key 3: The inertial factor

The natural tendency of any group of people is to resist change. It frequently helps those who are about to undergo a major change to talk with others who have recently made a similar change themselves. The best person to consult with about a pending change to a medical practice is another physician. Two ways to counteract inertia are:

- Select a role model for advice and leadership.

- Carry out an EMR transition in incremental steps. For example, begin with limited portions of the chart (medication and problem lists are the best candidates), follow with storage of dictation and transcription output, and add security measures later.

Automating a medical practice to the desired level of efficiency requires careful planning, consideration of many variables, and a sufficient allotment of time to complete. A practice cannot accomplish this assignment overnight. A successful system rollout can take two to three years, especially if the organization is a large, established practice with many paper charts.

To attain the solid support of users, EMR should do much more than simply serve as a powerful data storage and retrieval system. The electronic medical records system should be an integral part of the global management of the office. The fundamental reason for using EMR is its capabilities as a management and patient care tool.

One bona fide fear of moving to practice automation is that after spending time, effort, and expense, the medical practice will remain unimproved or even decline in efficiency. When an EMR system fails to meet expectations and provides fewer benefits than expected, it is often because users are not fully exploiting its features. Therefore, before implementing an EMR system, the physician and staff must identify specific operational areas that users expect EMR to improve. Once you install the system in the practice, you can measure its success against these established goals. The remaining sections of this chapter describe these operational areas.

The most obvious benefit of a computerized patient record system is that it provides the physician and staff with a neatly organized patient chart. This will benefit some practices more than others, depending on how well they currently maintain their records. Efficiencies and potential savings in this area will vary widely depending on the handwriting, dictating, and organizational skills of the people in each medical practice.

EMR as a Wise Investment

A recent report documenting the experiences of a group of medical clinics and practices that have been using EMR software developed a group of fourteen metrics with a focus on cost reduction, cost avoidance, and revenue improvement.[1] The user groups were diverse, representing both independent practices and those associated with and owned by large integrated delivery systems, and included both primary and specialty care facilities. They reported significant areas of financial benefit with EMR, including the following:

- Improved coding

- Labor savings

- Lower malpractice insurance premiums

- Reduced transcription expenses

Examples of benefits achieved include:

- In an integrated delivery system including forty-five clinics and more than 250 physicians, the implementation of EMR in just one clinic allowed for operation with two fewer staff positions for an annual savings of $60,000.

- In a six-physician clinic, as a result of higher productivity and improved coding, total charges billed per patient care increased 62.3 percent, from just over $89 to more than $145, in one year.

- In a specialty practice with nine physicians, malpractice insurance premiums decreased by $25,000 per year as a result of EMR improving documentation, reminders, and alerts.

- A solo urologist in private practice reported that EMR allows him to see 55-60 patients per day and has contributed to an 11 percent increase in charges per staff hour worked, while keeping the total number of staff hours worked 33 percent below the national benchmark for his specialty.

These results reflect the evaluation of clinic operation before the implementation of EMR and following 12 months of experience with the same software. Beyond confirming the hard-dollar potential, the evaluation also reveals a correlation between the value derived from EMR and the

---

1 *ROI: The White Paper*, developed by MedicaLogic, First Consulting Group and VHA, Inc.

length of use. As clinicians and staff become more comfortable with the system and as the EMR clinical database becomes fully populated, the full potential of workflow automation is realized.

Automating any business as intricate and complex as a medical practice requires a significant investment in time, materials, and cash flow. A natural question to ask before commencing with a project of this size is, "What is the expected return on our investment?" Answering this question involves taking an informed look at what EMR can do for the medical practice. It also requires an educated prediction about the promises future technologies might bring to your practice. We can classify most of the benefits associated with EMR in two ways:

- Cost reductions

- Opportunities for enhanced or improved patient care

Budgeting and Forecasting Investment Expenses

There is no doubt that computerizing the medical record requires a major initial expenditure. In practice, the initial purchase of computers and software should be treated as a usual capital budget, depreciable-over-five-years equipment purchase, since modern medical practice will increasingly demand at least some level of automation.

Budgeting should include the costs of software in addition to hardware purchases, as well. Pricing structures among software competitors vary, but typically incorporate a licensing fee per user. Also allow funds for maintenance; most vendors offer a yearly service contract that provides upgrades and renewable contracts for maintenance and support. You should plan to invest in upgrades or reconfigure your system, possibly even within several months after initial purchase and installation.

In addition to system equipment costs, also consider that computer systems consume time, paper, energy, space, and maintenance. In terms of cash management, treat the ongoing maintenance of EMR as an expense. This expense will be justified only if the tool provided is powerful, effective, and multifaceted. Any consideration of return on investment, therefore, should take into account all of the requirements of EMR and balance them with consideration of the following potential benefits:

Increased productivity. To what extent will your EMR allow you to see more patients in the same period?

- *Clinical data.* Clinicians save time with electronic medical records by more quickly accessing and reviewing patient records, documenting encounters, and communicating with other staff (by using flags). The immediate availability of important clinical data without time-consuming and error-prone redundant data entry can result in increased productivity, which can be quite profitable. If you can see one additional patient each half day, for example, because of the time EMR saves you, and your average total patient charge is $50, your yearly revenue will increase more than $25,000 per physician.

- *Scheduling.* If your EMR system is able to integrate with a scheduling tool, the physician gains more control over his or her time while staying focused on patients and patient records. This integration also enables greater teamwork by making the entire clinic's resources, staff, exam rooms, and equipment viewable from any authorized desktop.

- **Prescription writing.** A computerized medical record reduces or eliminates the need to write prescriptions. With EMR, physicians can simply print new prescriptions after updating the patient's medication list, combining two steps. This feature can save a physician five minutes or more for a patient with chronic conditions on multiple medications. The staff can then send prescription refill authorizations to pharmacies via fax modems, eliminating the need for manual paperwork and physical fax transmissions.

- **Automating referrals.** The EMR system also saves considerable time in automating referrals when it can transfer orders electronically between primary care physicians and specialists.

- **Utilization reviews.** EMR systems substantially reduce the time and cost of utilization reviews or quality-of-care reports, which we will cover extensively later in this chapter.

Market expansion. How can you use EMR to find new opportunities for expansion?

- **Direct contracting.** Suppose a local industry seeks a physician to perform a pre-employment physical. You should approach the prospective client with a well-planned and easy-to-understand business proposal, the first step to a long-term and mutually beneficial relationship.

  With your computer software program, you can develop a customized form containing all of the client's physical examination parameters. From your system, you can then automatically transmit copies of the completed form and any recommendations to the industry's business office on the same day you do the physical. No matter which office location the prospective employee uses, your standardized and customized exam will provide the client with the information they seek. This can be a powerful marketing tool for both individual practices and integrated health care systems.

- **Marketing to managed care companies.** Some EMR programs offer features that enable you to access clinical practice guidelines developed by expert panels of academic and practicing physicians. These clinical guidelines can save time for practitioners making referrals and may improve clinical decision-making at the point of care. Many MCOs like to see that physicians are incorporating clinical practice guidelines into their practice, because these MCOs see this as evidence of physicians striving for the most effective, efficient care.

Communicating with the patient. In the past, businesspeople compiled and typed mailing lists by hand on manual typewriters. Now, we take office automation for granted, and even people who work from offices in their homes have personal computers.

Medical office automation will most likely follow this pattern. In the coming years, medical office automation will be essential to keeping pace with the industry, and physicians will regard EMR as a cost of doing business.

- **Letters, forms, brochures, etc.** The physician will communicate with his patients as other businesses communicate, maximizing every aspect of office automation. Mass mailings to the community, computerized forms, letters to patients, E-mail interchanges, practice brochures, and advertising pieces are all possible applications of this EMR function.

- **Internet E-mail.** With the online services available through the Internet, your patients can communicate with you via E-mail. Typically, E-mail messages are brief and informal in structure and format, similar to a memorandum rather than a letter.

E-mail offers several distinct advantages. The patient can send messages to your office at his or her convenience, and you (or your staff) can reply at your convenience. When saved to a file, the E-mail message and your response can become a part of the patient's medical record. Usually, E-mail can reduce the number of phone calls you receive and return, as well as notes from staff members within your office. E-mail messages can also be forwarded to other members of your staff as appropriate, or to referring physicians, or when making referrals. Finally, E-mail can greatly decrease the number of "sticky notes" you use and perhaps even allay the concerns of the anxious patient.

Exhibit 1–2   E-Mail Screen

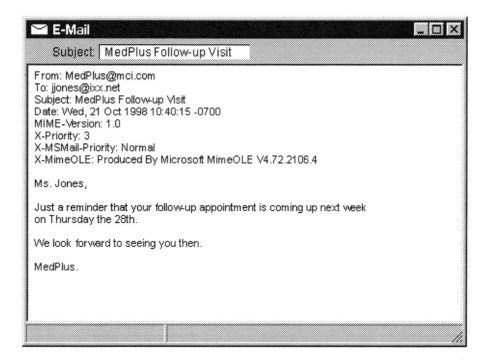

- *Internet as a health information resource.* Ours is an information-hungry society, and patients seek involvement in clinical decisions. You can help to expand your patients' understanding of their health by referring them to a web site that offers relevant information.

The Internet provides patient education resources on disease management (e.g., diabetes) and chat groups for individuals who share the same disorders. A computer terminal in your office that is available for your patients' use can enhance that patient's understanding and ease the tension that lack of understanding fosters.

Be sure you know the quality of the information you direct your patients to by checking your resources firsthand. Your health system may be a good resource for information on surgical procedures, and pharmaceutical companies may also sponsor reliable disease management information through the Internet.

Exhibit 1–3   **AMA Web Site**

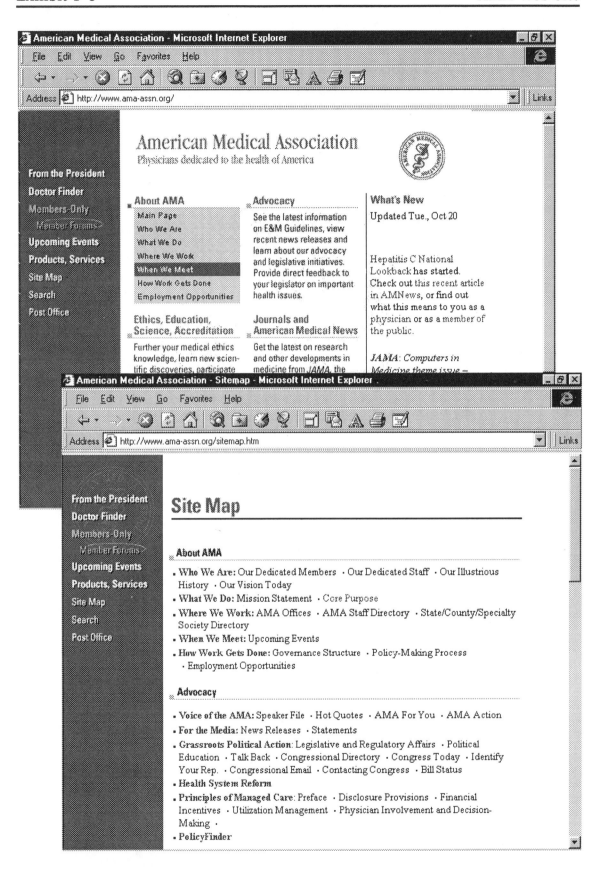

Exhibit 1–4   Health Information Resource

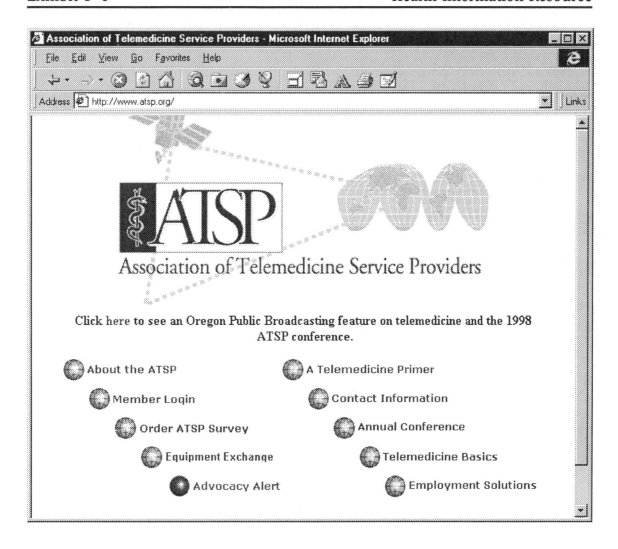

The resources available and the benefits that result will only increase as the Internet becomes familiar territory for the population at large. If you go to any major Internet search engine (Yahoo, Infoseek, or Search.com, for example), entire libraries of health care links are available.

Decreased costs. The following are concrete examples of how EMR can save money in salaries and overhead, both long-term and short-term.

- **Reduction in chart room storage.** Electronic record systems reduce the need for paper storage space considerably. Paper charts are necessary only for storing EKGs, x-rays, and similar items that cannot be easily stored electronically.

  Since the chart room in a mid-size to large clinic (e.g., fifty physicians) requires as much space as three exam rooms, which could support one revenue-generating clinician, EMR chart storage represents an opportunity cost of $200,000 to $300,000 per year.

- **Reduced chart pulls.** Other savings occur when the frequency of such functions as continuously pulling and refiling charts are decreased.

- *Improved cash flow.* Immediate access to information, simultaneously available to multiple users, can significantly reduce the time required to post a patient visit to the accounting system. Faster payment turnarounds, simplified by electronic billing (Electronic Data Interchange), improve cash flow in many ways.

First, having a medical record at the patients' point of entry and departure (the front office) allows information to be brought forth very quickly. Published estimates reveal that 3 to 15 percent of billings get lost between the delivery of services and the clinic's receipt of third-party payment. With EMR, no bill is ever held up because files are lost or in use. And, when a patient checks out, charges can be automatically tallied and copayments and deductibles collected before the patient leaves the office. The front office staff with access to EMR will have all relevant information necessary to determine what the patient owes, ensuring that reimbursement at the front end results in fewer charges that land in outstanding receivables.

Second, for balances owed after application of insurance payments, online information access allows the bill to be in the mail within two or three days.

Third, EMR information has greater integrity and is more likely to meet payer billing requirements. Payers often reject poorly documented bills and returning them to clinical business offices, where rejected claims require accounting representatives to engage in a time-consuming search for records to substantiate the billing, resubmit the bill, then wait for reimbursement (and perhaps a billing penalty). EMR systems help break the cycle.

Finally, electronic interfaces between EMR and your billing system speed up reimbursement from insurers. Claims filed electronically are paid much sooner than paper filings. Some carriers even transfer funds to your bank account via electronic funds transfer (EFT). In the recovery of funds, for every percent that the cash flow improves, each physician earns $2,000 to $3,000 annually.

- *Improved coding.* Improved coding of patient diagnoses result in more complete reimbursements. Under the old paper-based system, physicians wrote diagnoses directly on superbills, and staff members were later responsible for finding the correct diagnostic codes for reimbursement. Often, there was a high incidence of correct coding being lost in translation between the physician and the final billing.

EMR remedies this situation by removing the middle steps. A physician is able to immediately search and find the correct diagnostic codes while still in the exam room with the patient, increasing the accuracy and comprehensiveness of coding significantly.

- *Labor savings.* EMR allows for a smoother workflow and saves time for employees, who can be dedicated to other tasks. Among the greatest time savings for front-desk personnel is not having to return the numerous calls each week that require information from patient records. With that information available on-line, patient questions can usually be answered immediately. Clerical and clinical staff members also save time by not having to take and return calls from consulting physicians.

Your staff will spend less time on the telephone because of the speed with which they can take care of problems with patient information in front of them. Currently, in many practices, when patients call, the telephone receptionist takes their name and number and then pulls the chart. A staff member gives the chart to the nurse, who then calls back the patient when she gets time. Often with EMR, the nurse at a computer already has access to the patient's chart, and the receptionist can transfer the call directly without having to return a call. Time savings like these add up over a few days.

- ***Reducing staff and equipment.*** By decreasing the number of simple, repetitive tasks that the EMR now handles, larger offices may actually be able to cut staff. Small offices, while less likely to reduce staff, can achieve savings, reduce overhead, and create more room for efficiency, allotting more time for attention to other details.

  EMR may also reduce the number of telephone lines needed for your practice. With faster information processing, your patients should spend less time waiting on hold, freeing up your phone lines for incoming calls.

- ***Transcription savings.*** Computerized structured note forms for recording patient encounter information enable transcriptionists to work more efficiently. Many computer-literate physicians also enter their own chart notes into electronic records, virtually eliminating their transcription costs. Since most physicians spend from $300 to $2,000 per month on transcription, every 10 percent saved by EMR would reduce those costs by $360 to $2,400 annually.

- ***Storage and supplies.*** The computer will also save the expense of purchasing preprinted superbills. Instead, by printing out a record of the patient's charges by diagnosis and procedure codes, the need for storing forms is eliminated.

  Supply costs are also reduced as chart folders, dividers, and filing cabinets are used less by the practice. Practices using EMR also reduce the use of microfilm, paper, microfiche, copying, and off-site storage.

  Finally, rather than purchasing preprinted handouts, databases offer patient education and drug information handouts that can be printed on an as-needed basis. This reduces storage and waste, since you will use only as many handouts on asthma, for instance, as patients you see with asthma.

- ***Malpractice premium savings.*** Because of improved documentation and quality of care, malpractice insurers are beginning to reduce premiums for physicians using computerized patient record systems. Even a typical premium credit of 5 percent can save hundreds, or even thousands, of dollars per year for a physician.

- ***Patient relations.*** Another return on investment might result from providing better patient relations. Although a less tangible benefit than reduced costs, patient satisfaction has a significant impact on the practice.

  With EMR, medical staff are more aware of medical histories, and clinic staff are better able to communicate about lab test results, respond to telephone calls, accomodate medication and refill requests, and meet scheduled appointments. Finally, administrative staff members have more patient information at hand and can therefore interact more personably with the patients.

EMR as an Operations Management Tool

The priority for your use of EMR software is the same as all operations in your office, namely, the delivery of efficient, cost-effective health care. EMR should be an effective tool with which to review and evaluate your practice as a business operation, apart from the medical care you deliver. Maximizing efficiency in the daily flow of staff, patients, paper, and materials is the foremost reason to institute the use of EMR. Reducing the growing mountain of paperwork accompanying each health care visit might, alone, make this a worthwhile investment.

■ *Improving patient flow.* For most offices, a manager is in charge of the day-to-day operation of the office. This manager may report either to a larger entity, such as a hospital, or directly to the physician. In both cases, EMR provides an efficient conduit for communication and operational response. The office manager can see the "flow" of the office using the EMR software. If, for example, EMR tracks the time a patient arrives, the manager can quickly determine how well the front office is keeping up with the patient flow. If a backlog occurs, the manager can query staff members through the computer terminal and immediately adjust workflow and assignments.

■ *Meeting operational benchmarks.* The ability to keep tabs on up-to-the-minute operational benchmarks makes your office manager efficient and powerful. In integrated health care systems, it is the office manager who functions as a liaison between corporate policy and operational flow. Using EMR, the manager can institute policy by using templates and electronic memos.

■ *Improving interoffice communications.* When the receptionist receives a telephone call for a physician from the emergency room, normally he or she must find the physician to take the call immediately. Using the capability of some EMR software, the receptionist can easily track a physician's location within the clinic by determining which computer the physician is using, then transferring the call directly without asking, paging, or getting out of the chair. This allows the receptionist to spend more time processing and caring for patients and reduces instances of a patient approaching the front desk only to find no one there. Always having someone available at the front desk will decrease frustration and improve patient satisfaction, an increasingly important benchmark for managed care.

The fact that everyone in the office routinely uses a computer also enables instant communication. Interoffice E-mail can greatly reduce the time spent communicating. Being able to electronically attach a message to a patient's chart means that tasks or problems with patients can be directed appropriately at any time. These tasks will then remain a part of the recipient's electronic desktop until the staff member resolves the matter. This electronic message feature eliminates time lost searching for a message buried under a stack of charts on the desk. Also, archaic phrases like, "We can't find the chart" and "I didn't get your message" no longer apply. The computer can organize each employee's work duties by taking over time- and space-management tasks.

■ *Managing staff objectively.* Using comparative data, you and your office manager can more objectively evaluate the job your staff is doing. For example, if the requirements for nurse charting are increasing, especially in the outpatient setting, you need to know that your nurse is fulfilling these requirements. EMR allows you to generate customized reports, based on your criteria, that can function as a basis for making a judgment. Asking the EMR database to return all charts with tetanus shots given by Nurse A, separate from Nurse B, for instance, can simplify a chart audit comparing the nurse with the standard.

Conversely, you can convert a performance standard into an efficient tool for the nurse. Every year, you may give many patients influenza shots, and all of the shots generally come from the same batch and have the same expiration date and lot number. You instruct the responsible nurse to chart all of this information. With EMR, your nurse or system administrator can program a "hot key" that charts the shot with a single keystroke.

These abilities to evaluate, react to and improve the operation of your practice make EMR an asset with value far greater than a neatly organized chart.

EMR as a Patient Care Tool

One of the most often-voiced fears about EMR from physicians is that having a computer terminal in the exam room will somehow interfere with the patient-physician relationship. On the contrary, however, patients are familiar with computers in every aspect of their lives. The fact that their chart is electronic, and that computers are part of their health care support, will come as no surprise. Increasing numbers of the population have home computers, and most of their jobs are done with some assistance from computers. Considering the computer's routine presence in both businesses and homes, its acceptance in the exam room is likely to be quite high. (Still, the physician may have to put up with routine jokes about computers replacing bad handwriting.)

Data gathered from patients suggest strong patient acceptance of, and support for, computerized patient records. A recent study found that[2]:

■ Sixty-four percent of the patients whose healthcare providers had implemented EMR believed that the quality of their care has improved because of the system.

■ Twenty-nine percent reported no change.

■ The remaining 7 percent had no opinion or believed the quality of care had declined.

■ Sixty percent indicated that the quality of service they receive has improved, with 28 percent seeing no change, and the remaining 12 percent not offering an opinion or seeing a reduction.

Portable options such as notebook computers and Personal Digital Assistants (PDAs) even allow physicians to hold the computers in their laps much like the familiar paper record, easing the transition between the two record systems.

■ *Improving medical charts.* Medical charts have always had a mysterious quality to them. Patients are quite naturally curious to know exactly what the physician is writing, especially since the medical record is a permanent, private document. Having this information available in the exam room gives your medical record system an open, honest quality that is much appreciated by patients. Seeing their medical chart summarized on the computer screen may also help to prompt their memory, which can stimulate more comprehensive answers to your questions.

■ *Streamlining patient care standards and guidelines.* EMR provides a quality patient care tool because it can instantly "remember" and find database information one would normally have to memorize or look up manually. It can also prompt physicians and staff to remember designated procedures or policies. This becomes especially important in managed care settings.

---

1 Conducted by Griggs Anderson Research and MedicaLogic.

If, for example, an organization agrees to adhere to certain patient care standards, a system administrator can input these standards using a template and distribute them to all of the participating clinics. In such a case, the physician can evaluate the care of a patient with "new onset diabetes" against a standard template that can prompt everything from education on foot care to necessary laboratory work. EMR can also prompt follow-up visits and track health maintenance items. Many databases are available commercially or can be customized by your health care organization. Following are some examples:

- Patient information handouts

- Pharmaceutical databases, including checking for drug-drug interaction

- HMO and PPO rules, provider panels, and formularies

- Diagnosis and procedure coding

- Customized orders for inpatient and outpatient procedures ordered elsewhere

- Lab reference values

- Algorithms for diagnostic work-ups

In the study cited above, 74 percent of practices using EMR reported that the quality of the service they deliver had improved, and 63 percent reported an improvement in the quality of their work life.

Exhibit 1-5   Patient Education and Information Software

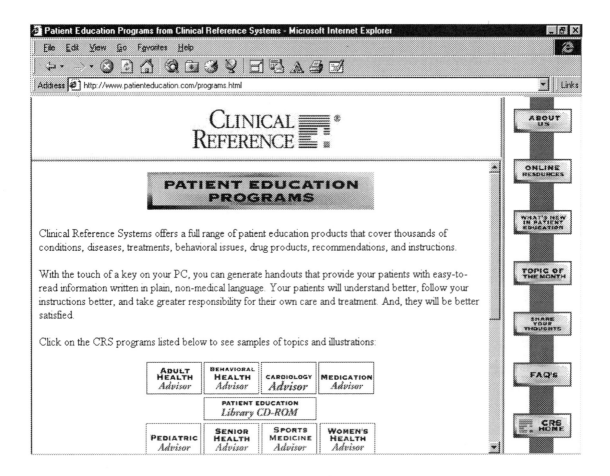

- *Personalizing patient care.* EMR supports a personalized approach to patient care. You can chart and print for the patient individual data, such as blood pressure readings, blood sugars, and other customized handouts. Seeing a printed chart of increasing blood sugars with his or her name on it can be a powerful motivating agent for a patient's self-care, demonstrating your individualized treatment for them and reinforcing the idea of personalized care.

  A good EMR will also provide patient identification cards that include allergies, medications, and advance care directives. This feature may hasten or improve care in an emergency room setting or if the patient is seeking care while traveling.

- *Streamlining patient referrals.* You can also expect that the quality of referred patient care will rise dramatically with EMR, even if the referral doctor is not on the same system as you. Generating a copy of the chart is as easy as a keystroke, and copies can be prepared for the patient to take with him or her, if necessary. In fact, you can fax entire charts to referral doctors more quickly than you used to be able to reach them by telephone.

Another scenario that makes the physician appreciate EMR is the middle-of-the-night telephone call from the emergency room. If the ER notifies you at 3:00 a.m. that your patient needs urgent surgery and the surgeon needs the patient's medical background, you can access the patient chart housed in your office by using your home computer (or laptop) and a modem. You can then direct your office system to transmit the chart, via fax, directly to the emergency room. The result is efficient patient care using accurate information, and more sleep and rest for you!

Exhibit 1-6   Patient Care (i.e., visit to a radiology home page to learn about MRIs)

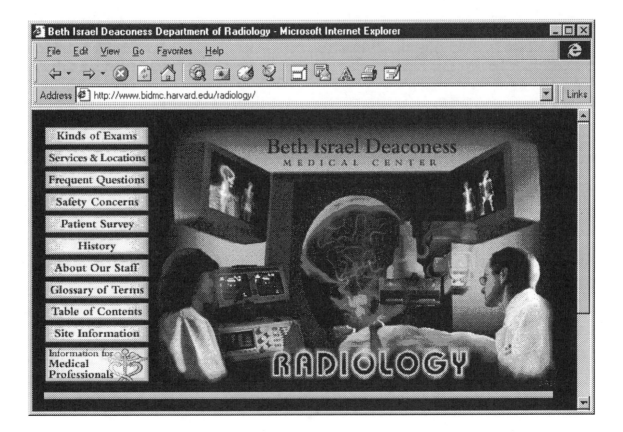

EMR as a Patient Record

A patient record is a place to store information that is ultimately available for many purposes other than direct medical care. EMR allows the user to retrieve information usefully and reproducibly, and its ability to present aggregate data is an impelling tool for purposes such as utilization review, medical research and the development of patient care pathways. Still, EMR also contributes significant day-to-day advantages as a patient record.

- *Chart review.* Typically, paper charts are placed in a chart rack outside the exam room door, where the physician examines its contents for a few seconds before entering the room to see the patient. The merit of this brief review is directly proportional to the organization of the chart. In contrast, EMR permits a physician to review an entire day's worth of patients while having a cup of coffee in the morning, and all of the information will be organized uniformly and consistently for every patient.

- *Problem lists.* With EMR, problem lists are easily kept up-to-date, medications organized, and labs reviewed using a flowchart instead of a thick sheaf of reports.

- *Practice profile.* EMR allows each physician to view a profile of his or her practice at any time. This information can be useful in positioning for managed care contracts, predicting future growth, or viewing medical practice decisions made over prior periods. If your accountant tells you that you can discount only a certain percentage of your practice to managed care, for instance, you should expect that office automation has tracked this for you.

Exhibit 1-7   Patient Record (i.e., another excerpt from Mrs. Jones's chart)

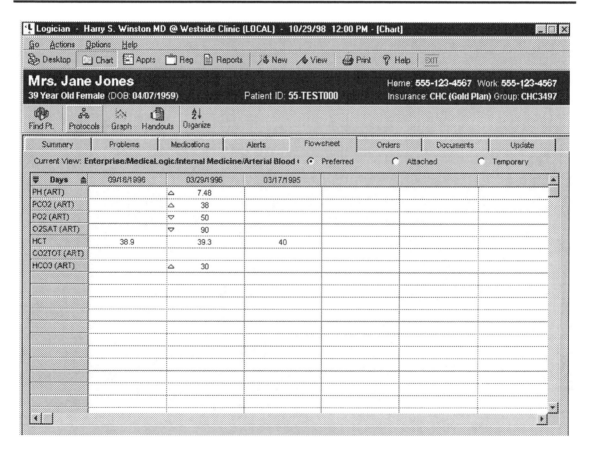

EMR as a Support to Employees

Far too often, when patients call a medical office, the first thing they hear is, "good morning, can I put you on hold?" The caller's immediate impression may be that the office is overwhelmed, understaffed, and unable to care for patients. The receptionist who has answered the telephone, spoken to a patient, then placed the call on hold does not yet know what the patient wants and has to answer the telephone again, doubling the number of times she or he answers the telephone. Moreover, the patient may be annoyed.

- *Improving telephone support.* EMR can rectify the twice-answered telephone situation. By empowering the employee and providing the tools to route patient calls, EMR lets the receptionist take care of the patient during the few seconds he or she would normally place the caller on hold.

  Sometimes, of course, patients may still be placed on hold after they have stated their needs, but their waiting time will be shortened by EMR. This routine will decrease the frustration levels of both the receptionist and the patient.

- *Improving employee performance.* EMR will better equip employees to handle their job functions, and they will know they are good at their jobs. Because EMR documents employee activities, the physician can use that information as a motivational tool to give routine positive feedback to staff. Since employee turnover is one of the great hidden costs to a business, an increase in employee satisfaction is sure to pay long-term dividends.

Providing Care to Another Physician's Patients

Having tests available with names of the people who administered them comes in handy when you see your partners' patients in your practice. A physician covering for a colleague in an automated office will no longer have difficulty locating misplaced or recently delivered lab results, for example, since they will already have been delivered directly into the electronic medical record. Finding such information as routine urinalysis documentation is as simple as entering the patient name, with all other information being handled by the EMR. The covering physician can then easily edit records and enter results directly into the computer in the order of the dipstick results. (See Exhibit 1–8 for example.)

Exhibit 1-8　　　　　　　　　　　　　　　　　　　**Lab Work, Urinalysis**

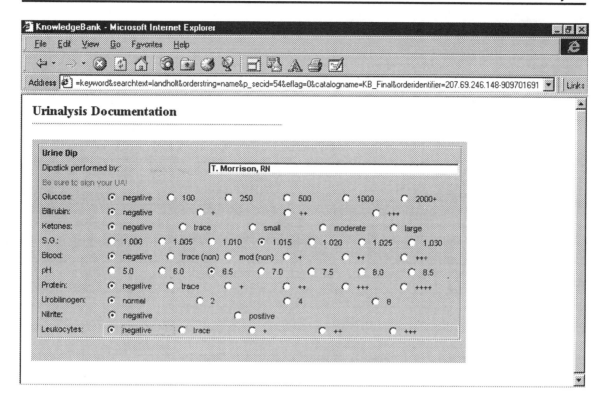

EMR as a Risk-Management Tool

Electronic medical records are having a significant impact on malpractice premiums nationwide. Some malpractice insurance carriers, for instance, certify certain existing software for discounts because the electronic medical record eliminates the potential for challenges to vague, questionable handwriting in a court of law (a common area of dispute for paper records). EMR also helps to manage risk in other significant ways.

- *Providing reliable reporting.* EMR enables the generation of reliable, reproducible reports on the proper documentation of care. Health care systems, therefore, can easily evaluate a physician's performance compared with established standards or other physicians. With a high level of confidence in the quality of care the physician constituents deliver, confirmed by data derived from EMR reporting mechanisms, some health systems are willing to self-insure with secondary stop-loss insurance, thereby assuming increased financial risk.

- *Meeting accrediting agency standards (NCQA, HEDIS 3.0, JCAHO, OSHA, etc.).* Accrediting agencies are increasing attention to outpatient activities. JCAHO and HCFA standards do not, for instance, allow physicians to sign notes without reviewing the content of the record. The use of electronic medical records easily encourages proper behavior by alerting staff to standard options of operation. While the systems will not mandate behavior or override a physician's ability to choose nonstandard options for care, the EMR system will automatically document behavior and adherence to the standard without need for further review or discussion. For example, medication and problem lists, allergies, and directives such as DNR orders are part of the program code of EMR and are automatic functions. This application eliminates much of the stress, time, and resources health care systems expend preparing for review or accreditation.

Making Occupational Safety and Health Administration (OSHA) standards and procedures regular parts of the record reduces the burden of documenting for OSHA requirements. A good example is documentation for urinalysis done in the office. EMR automatically enters the names of the people who performed the test.

- **Preparing for practice audits.** Today's medical offices, especially if they are part of an integrated health system, have a seemingly endless stream of visitors who arrive onsite with a checklist of some kind. Various utilization reviewers, Joint Commission on Accreditation of Healthcare Organizations (JCAHO) inspectors, and Medicare auditors are among those who have an agenda for auditing your practice.

Besides placing a burden on your staff to furnish information, inquiries disrupt the operation of the office itself when physicians and staff must divert their time, effort, energy, space, and other attentions from patient care in order to satisfy these auditing requirements. It is in everyone's best interest that reviewers perform their jobs quickly and easily, allowing the office to return as quickly as possible to concentrating on its primary function, which is patient care. An EMR system helps your staff provide the necessary information quickly and simplifies the reviewer's job. With easily attained data, your office staff makes a positive impression on the auditor.

The JCAHO reviewer has a typical checklist to complete when performing a practice audit. The EMR can help in two ways:

1. **Compliance.** Since functions are automatic, the record will comply with the standard of care.

   A prime example is the *problem list*. By its program codes, EMR software presents an easily identifiable problem list, including corresponding diagnostic (ICD-9) codes to comply with the standard of care for those symptoms the patient exhibits.

   For example, if a patient presents with elevated blood pressure (140 over 100), the blood pressure reading can be entered directly into the EMR and compared to previous readings, since the flowsheet automatically records new data next to previously recorded data. In the diagnosis section, the physician enters *hypertension* and gets all applicable ICD-9 codes for high blood pressure. When *Essential Hypertension 401.9* is chosen, the code is automatically entered into the problem list. Prescribed medication is likewise recorded in the medication list, which automatically gives the physician a running list of all previous medications, side effects, etc.

2. **Functionality.** The EMR makes certain functions easy to perform.

   To check drug-drug interaction, for instance, a good EMR system has a database that enables comparison of all medications and allergies in a patient's record. If this function is easy to use and if it documents the provider's due diligence in checking, the physician is certain to use it. A reviewer can easily audit this function and document his or her findings. The physician who maintains these documentation habits is cast in a positive light without expending anyone's additional time or effort. As automation evolves, the frequency of JCAHO and similar audits should diminish or disappear.

The following checklist outlines some medical chart standards required by organizations such as National Commission on Quality Assurance (NCQA) and JCAHO. We have organized the list according to record content, maintenance, and medical care information. The level of assistance provided by EMR for meeting standards follows each item.

One property to look for in EMR software is flexibility with regard to particular physician behavior. The system must not require him or her, for instance, to fill out certain predetermined care plans, e.g., return visits; these recommendations may change for each patient. Be sure that the EMR's automatic functions do not interfere with the physician's decision-making. In no way should a feature force a physician to behave in a certain way while he or she is taking care of patients.

NCQA and JCAHO Standards Checklist

Following is a general checklist for physician organizations seeking to meet medical record standards set by NCQA and JCAHO. The purpose of this list, obtained from these accreditors, is to illustrate the value of electronic medical records in helping the physician meet quality standards.

Record Content

1. Formats of record keeping are standardized within a health care system.

   Standard formats are an automatic function of EMR software.

2. All entries are dated and legible.

   Dated and legible entries are an automatic function of EMR software.

3. All pages of the record identify the patient.

   Record ID is an automatic function of EMR software.

4. Only authorized individuals make entries.

   The EMR assists this practice because the record defines levels of participation. For example, a front-office staff member does not have necessary access to the patient record to prescribe a medication.

5. Provider is easily identified; each entry is identified by person making entry and authenticated by signature or initials.

   The provider's identification is an automatic function of EMR software. Courts of law recognize electronic signatures as legal.

6. Verbal orders are accepted/transcribed.

   EMR assists this function because the software automatically identifies the person accepting the order.

7. Summary list is present in the chart for diagnoses, symptoms, allergies, adverse reactions, and medications. The list must be developed on or before third visit and must be found in the same area of the chart.

   These lists are automatic functions of EMR. This record-keeping capability exceeds standards because lists are always present at the first visit.

8. Records contain health maintenance flowsheet, social and family history, and immunization records.

   This function can be automatic; however, each practice might need to input customized forms for its specialty or focus (e.g., a pediatrician would customize his or her practice's immunization records differently than a geriatrician).

9. Documentation of smoking habits, alcohol use, substance abuse is present.

   Use of customized forms and ease of input assists in this documentation process. The function is not necessarily automatic.

10. Plans for return visits or other follow-up activities are documented.

    EMR can help with this documentation, although the function is not automatic.

11. Consultation, laboratory, and x-ray reports are filed promptly after being initialed by physician.

    Currently, EMR does not generally assist this function since the practice must store these in a paper chart. As scanning devices and technologies improve, the mechanism for filing paper reports will also improve, as explained elsewhere in this book. (See Chapter 3, page 43.)

12. Record contains explicit notation and documentation of abnormal results/patient notification/patient recall.

    Ease of entry assists this routine somewhat. It is partially automatic by use of automatic notification systems.

13. Coding of diagnoses and procedures to meet ICD-9, CPT, or other standardized nomenclatures.

    This is an automatic function of EMR.

14. All terminologies, definitions, vocabularies, abbreviations, and symbols are standard throughout the medical record.

    EMR's capacity to store lists of information for use at the time of the encounter assists in meeting this standard. These lists can prompt appropriate usage by the person entering the data.

Record Maintenance

1. The retention of medical records is standardized within the department.

   This is an automatic process of EMR.

2. Medical records are completed within 14 days of the visit.

   EMR assists this practice by ease of record entry for all visits. EMR automatically exceeds the standard for many visits since the caregiver will complete some record entries before the patient leaves the exam room!

3. Practitioners are not permitted to remove medical records from office.

EMR exceeds the standard by never allowing the physician to "remove" the record, yet the physician can work on charting from home through remote access. EMR simultaneously allows security and availability of data.

4. Medical records are secured by locked storage.

This measure is an automatic feature of EMR by means of electronic security.

5. Records are protected always against loss, destruction, or unauthorized use.

This protection is an automatic function of EMR. It exceeds the standard by allowing backup tapes to be kept offsite, allowing restoration of records even if a fire (or other comparable disaster) destroys the practice facility.

6. Special security arrangements are made for confidential charts.

Security is an automatic feature of EMR and is addressed through the establishment of access hierarchies.

7. Department policy to review ambulatory medical records for compliance is followed.

Other than ease of review, EMR offers no assistance in this routine. However, only those items that are not automatic need review.

8. Records are shared within the health care system to meet the medical needs of the patient.

This practice is automatic if the health care system uses a central database. Otherwise, EMR assists the process through its ease of printing and faxing records directly from computer system.

9. Uniform policy is in place for release of medical records, including electronic distribution of data.

EMR's capacity to store and print release forms assists with this function.

Medical Care Information

1. Diagnosis is consistent with the findings.

Ease of searching ICD-9 codes assists with this practice.

2. Plans for action and treatment are consistent with findings.

Use of standardized forms for certain types of visits assists in this routine (e.g., a standard UTI visit filled out on the screen is designed to satisfy this requirement, if filled out appropriately).

3. Consultants are used appropriately to avoid under- and overutilization.

EMR does not offer assistance in this area other than documenting the information for study, which can be used later as a tool for change.

4. Continuity of care, coordination, and communication between primary and specialty physicians is evidenced.

   EMR does not offer assistance in this area other than in its ability to document telephone calls. However, if the health care system is on a wide area network (WAN), it may be possible that the primary and specialty care physicians are actually using the same charts. This centralized database will allow a practice to demonstrate continuity of care between the primary and specialty care physicians.

5. Care appears to be medically appropriate; laboratory and other diagnostic studies are ordered as appropriate.

   EMR assists somewhat, through its ability both to list allowable codes for certain procedures and to make the medical record available for physician review during the encounter.

6. Evidence is presented that preventive screening is offered using protocols and reminders.

   Parts of this function are automatic but require input of care providers to set protocols, timing of reminders, etc. Ease of generating letters, labels, and custom lists makes the process virtually automatic.

EMR as Part of Information Systems

Most software programs offer fully integrated electronic medical records and practice management modules to form a combined information system. These programs also support communication with other information systems (e.g., other offices, labs, hospitals) but often require an interface application.

As an example, a unified health care organization purchases and installs a superb EMR system, and it works well—perhaps even better than expected. At the end of the day, the system furnishes the medical office a report containing the complete CPT and ICD-9 codes needed for billing. However, the EMR and billing system can not "talk" to each other. Without an interface application, which acts as a translator between the two systems, the office billing staff must manually enter paper batches of superbills into the billing system.

- *Interfacing systems.* This points out the need for "interfacing" or "integrating." Interface engines are a combination of software and hardware designed to make disparate software systems communicate meaningfully.

- *System compatibility.* Beyond considering the compatibility of software and hardware, you must also consider whether the supplying companies themselves are compatible. For interface engines to do their job, all of the vendors whose software/hardware is involved must be willing to work together to make the interface work reliably.

  The medical computer industry recognizes the importance of interfacing and is striving to provide solutions that ensure its aggregate technical problems do not become the clinical problems of its physician customers. The Andover Group, for example, is a council of technical experts from a variety of software and hardware companies (many of whom are competitors) whose mission is to develop a set of networking standards specific to the needs and wants of the health care industry. The Andover Group will build on existing standards to attack the most oft-cited ailment in health care information management: lack of compatibility among information systems.

- *Billing systems—handling demographic information.* Most medical practices have an automated billing system in place when they convert to computerized medical records. Ideally, the billing system should present patient demographic data with the electronic medical record, which eliminates the need to reenter this information into the patient's chart.

  If, for example, your office signs up one hundred new patients from a managed care organization, which electronically sends you the demographic information on these patients, your system should then allow you to download it into your database and share the data between EMR and billing modules of the systems.

- *Laboratory software.* Tracking and follow-up of lab reports has always been complex, and getting laboratory results into your chart can be a time-consuming process. Electronic medical records eliminate this hassle when an interface exists between the EMR and lab software systems.

  The electronic automation of lab values is a two-way street. In an electronic system, labs are ordered from the chart and the appropriate results registered to the same chart without the need to manually fill out a single form. Users of these systems must be sure a reliable interface exists between the two vendors (i.e., EMR and laboratory).

  Interfacing is especially critical with hospital laboratories. Most hospital information systems are proprietary; that is, hospitals have programmers who write software for their mainframe computer(s) to care for all of its automation needs. These programmers are very knowledgeable and competent professionals who will need to understand your desire to "integrate" their technology with a commercial, PC-based product.

  Lab systems deal with result codes, a unique identifier for every lab test performed. These identifiers ensure that TSH and hTSH, for instance, find their way to the correct slot in the patient's EMR lab flowsheet. To properly integrate, the two components (the hospital programmers and the commercial PC-based product) must negotiate the master tables with code results. Standards are yet to be determined.

  Likewise, the hospital's system and the physician's EMR software must address platforms and other methods of computer communication. This requires the identification and assignment of responsibility to individuals in both systems who will solve future problems. The physician, though not usually knowledgeable of technical workings, must be aware of the processes needed to keep office automation smooth and efficient.

  Once lab values are in the electronic medical record, the physician has instant access to data. He or she can manipulate these data in any manner, including the generation of graphs.

- *Managed care software.* The development of managed care software presents the ultimate challenge for the computer industry. Managed care contracts touch every aspect of a health care delivery system. Labs, fee schedules, diagnoses, procedures, referrals, forms, reports, scheduling, and even educational activities can figure into a massive formula for reimbursement of the physician or health care system. Managed care arrangements require providers to follow multiple layers of rules. For patients in capitated plans, the physician sometimes receives monies without ever seeing the patient. Keeping track of the massive flow of information is complicated and time-consuming.

Managed care software is designed to handle many billing and reimbursement issues. Ultimately, automation of the entire process requires the development of an interface that enables communication with every aspect of your practice. The accomplishment of this technical challenge will herald the advent of the totally integrated medical practice.

- **Communications, faxes, and E-mail.** The seamless flow of communication is critical in the delivery of health care, and for best results, the flow must be seamless.

  - **Faxes.** Facsimile transmission is used routinely in medical practices. Most practices use fax machines (desktop equipment designed to send and receive facsimiles over telephone lines) to transmit copies of documents from one location to another. To transmit patient information by a fax machine, usually a staff member must copy material from the chart, generate a typed letter, and then manually place the papers on a fax machine.

  - **Text recognition.** A more seamless way to send patient information is by using the text recognition capabilities of the EMR system. These technologies, as integral parts of the system, allow you to eliminate paper when faxing. The sender electronically transfers all pertinent data to the receiver, whether these are phone messages, faxes, paging, E-mail, etc. These communiqués then automatically become part of the medical record.

  - **E-mail.** An efficient, timesaving, and cost-effective tool for communication, E-mail permits you to send a message anywhere in the world without incurring a charge for postage or long distance service. The delivery is almost instantaneous and is highly reliable. Many health care systems now have local E-mail capabilities (using an Intranet) within their own mainframe system for interoffice communication. Some systems are building electronic links for communication over the Internet.

The marriage of these communication technologies will enable physicians to communicate promptly and efficiently with other practices. When a physician in a small town refers a patient to a metropolitan-area specialist, he or she can send a letter by E-mail with the patient's chart attached as an electronic file. With a proper interface, the specialist can then place the file into his or her computer system and append it accordingly. He or she then reverses the process by updating the primary physician's EMR with all of the new information.

Vendors have taken steps to ensure security and confidentiality for the future. The delivery of health care to the patient improves because of the instant availability of information.

Exhibit 1-9   Drug Information Software, Drug-Drug Interaction Warning

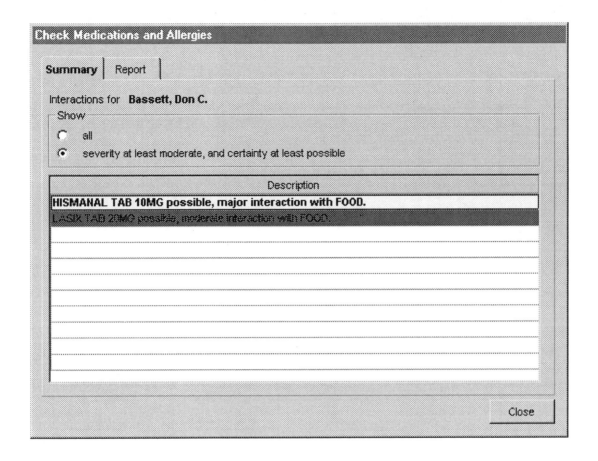

Moving Forward with EMR

Overall, when most physicians weigh the potential costs and benefits of EMR, they realize that their practices will gain substantially from at least some level of automation. The rapid spread of computer technology promises to eventually make traditional charting and record keeping a thing of the past, and EMR is likely to become as indispensable to medical practice as x-rays, lasers, and magnetic resonance imaging. That being the case, the most likely question for a physician to ask is not whether to implement EMR, but when and how to move forward with office automation. The next two chapters include information that will help you begin forming answers to those questions.

CHAPTER 2

Preparing the Office for Transition

Considering the Cost

The cost for implementing an electronic medical records system must fit within the budget of your practice. The size and scope of the project involves the following parameters:

- Number of workstations

- Size of the network

- Number and kinds of software the network is able to run

- Amount of training that can be afforded prior to purchasing the EMR system

- Cost of maintaining a system (which is significant)

Initially, most physicians want to select top-of-the-line systems and software, but they sometimes find these do not fit their budget. Instead of overextending, you may want to scale back on features and options and make plans to expand and enhance the system in the future.

Prior to purchase, you should set up demonstrations of the software packages you are considering. Allow administrative and clinical staff to get hands-on experience before making the final decision. Staff members like receptionists and nurses will then be equipped to ask vendors pointed questions about how the product will change your practice operation.

Although the package you can afford may not be all you want, the staff will gain expertise by using the equipment and evaluating its use. This background will be useful for future training and staff development.

Buying or Leasing Equipment

Preparing for implementation begins with making the financial arrangements necessary to acquire your equipment. The investment is substantial, for both small and large practices. First, investigate whether to lease or buy a computer system. Ask your accountant to work out the numbers and to recommend a lease or purchase based on your total financial picture. Due to the rapid changes in technology, leases that allow upgrades and add-ons usually work well.

Phasing in the Changeover

Changeovers from manual systems to computerized functions are significant in small offices and even more difficult to accomplish in larger practices. Small practices often adapt to changeovers more readily because the physician generally has good control over the practice operations. An eight-physician practice with an entire staff count of 44, a large number of charts, multiple specialties, and various people using the charts may be most successfully brought on-line in phases. You may also have to develop a strategy for phasing in the computers themselves to minimize disruption.

While you are evaluating what kind of systems and software to buy, and while you are considering the purchase of a larger server and more computers, you should also develop a strategy that will allow you to change over in phases. Success usually results when one or two users become familiar with the system, work out the kinks with the vendor, and can support new uses as they are added incrementally.

When a changeover comes overnight, chaos almost always occurs, unless a great deal of preparation, training, and expertise are available on-site. For best results in converting a health system to computerized medical records, bring in small clusters of doctors and expand the technology as equipment is installed and people receive training.

Assembling Your Implementation Team

Many responsibilities and tasks are involved in implementing any new computer system. Selecting the right person to oversee the purchase and start-up is critical to deriving long-term success with EMR.

The networks necessary to run computers require routine and competent care. Because network experts are in short supply, one would not expect to find this level of knowledge from an employee in a typical medical office. Identifying and training a key person on your staff—or, in a larger practice, hiring an expert network administrator—to be responsible for the ongoing administration of your computer system is essential to success.

Begin by making an inventory of your own staff and evaluating each member's current knowledge and expertise in computer usage, as well as their demonstrated aptitude for mastering technology. Ideally, your office manager will have a high level of proficiency with computers and office automation; however, in many practices, another employee's skills may exceed those of the office manager. Identifying potential role conflicts prior to installing a computer system and resolving them in advance will help to prevent employee dissatisfaction that may arise over time.

Whether you are a one-physician office or part of a large health care organization, a team effort is necessary for successful implementation. Develop and maintain a master checklist designating tasks, responsibilities, completion dates, inventory lists, etc. Hold regular meetings to update the checklist and discuss any problems (schedule these at least weekly in the early phases of changeover preparation, daily when you get closer to your "go-live" date). Keep the checklist flexible enough to adapt to situations that may suddenly arise.

Finally, be sure to adjust pay levels and revise job descriptions for those asked to coordinate the computers in the office and to whom you assign additional responsibilities. Pay levels must correlate with expertise and responsibility.

Evaluating Your Workflow

Implementing computerized medical records and other components of office automation requires an early and critical look at exactly how your office functions. Computerized tools can have a positive impact on every aspect of your operation, and studying your current practice from a variety of viewpoints will allow you to see the full potential of office automation as it applies to your practice.

- *Examine your floor plan.* One important area to view closely is your physical layout and how it relates to patient encounters. Examination of the floor plan and physical movements of the patients and staff is the first step to understanding your workflow.

  Using a copy of your floor plan and colored pens, trace the physical movement for each person involved in a typical patient encounter. For instance, the patient line should start at the front door, go to the reception desk, then to the waiting area, back to the vital signs area, to an exam room, then back to the front desk. The patient's line would intersect with the nurse's line at the door to the exam rooms, for example.

  After you trace the lines for the physician, the nurse, the patient, the front office staff, the lab technicians, and others, look at the paths. If you find that your nurse, who probably performs the most physical tasks in your practice, has a long and circuitous route with every patient, you might consider changing the floor plan and/or finding a way to use your computers for some of these functions.

- *Perform time and motion studies.* One application of modifying workflow might be in sending fax transmissions. If your nurse has to fax referral forms to comply with a managed care contract but does not have easy access to a fax machine, consider your alternatives for alleviating the problem. Options might be adding another fax machine, adding a door for easier access, installing a fax server on your computer network so the nurse can fax the form from the computer file, or perhaps all three.

  One motive for purchasing an EMR system is to automate many tasks performed in each patient encounter. List every possible task performed in your office and who does it. The list will be lengthy, with multiple performers for many tasks. The list will give you an idea, from a time and motion standpoint, of who does the most work in your office. Generally, you will find that physicians perform the least number of physical tasks per patient visit. Your EMR system will initially benefit your staff more than it will benefit you, but as their efficiency increases, yours will also.

- *Review patient encounters.* Finally, examine how you see patients within the office. The workflow should feel comfortable and appropriate to the goals of your practice.

Taking a critical look at all aspects of your workflow while implementing your EMR will allow you to make long-term substantive changes that will benefit your practice in many ways throughout the years.

Wiring the Office and Locating Workstations

The more computers you have, the more expensive your conversion investment will be. A thorough examination of your practice workflow will help you decide on the proper number and locations for your computers. Execute your action plan as follows:

- *Determine how many stations you need.* The first task is deciding how many computers should make up your system. In a high-volume practice like pediatrics, a physician needs a terminal in each exam room to be the most efficient. More specialized practices with fewer patient visits may decide to keep the computers outside the exam room and print visit forms from the computer for the physician to use. Some physicians even choose to keep a full paper chart backup printed from the EMR; since all the computers are in the front office, their day-to-day practice does not change at all.

- *Plan terminal placements.* Next, you must decide where to place the computers (each individual screen and keyboard combination throughout the office is a separate "terminal"). Most terminals can be kept on a small counter, perhaps fifteen by thirty inches. Keyboards can be placed on a sliding drawer, out of sight and out of reach for small, busy hands of children. The central processing unit (CPU), the most expensive and important component of each computer, can be kept under a counter or mounted in a box on a wall.

  Within each exam room, choose the exact location of the computer station. This may depend on several parameters and your practice style. Some physicians like to look at the computer with the patient and locate the terminal conveniently for this purpose. Some internists wish to see the computer during the physical exam and keep it next to the examination table. Take your own preferences and practices into account during this stage of planning.

- *Design your wiring scheme.* Plan the computer wiring scheme of the office well ahead of the "go-live" date. Wiring requirements depend on the size and type of system you are purchasing. (More information on wiring is presented in *Chapter 3, Becoming Familiar with Computer Terminology.*) Wiring is a necessary and intrusive process, but having the wiring thoroughly tested for reliability before attaching any computers to it is vitally important.

Surveying Training Needs

Your practice may need computer training on several levels. Some of your employees may be very familiar with using computers through various functions of their jobs, while others may have almost no experience. You may be moving from a DOS-based program to a Windows® environment. If your new computerized medical records system is a Windows®-based program, you can arrange basic Windows® and mouse training through a local computer company. You should schedule additional training for medical records software, word processing, faxing, and any other programs you plan to use. The goal is to bring all the staff, including the physicians, up to the knowledge level at which they can function comfortably using the computer system and software.

Training to use and care for the terminals and printers is a separate issue from training to use EMR software applications. The software and hardware vendors whom you select can help you develop a list of do's and don'ts for system management within the office. These guidelines will facilitate the use of the system and help you to avoid problems down the road.

- ***Set up guidelines.*** Protect your system by having routines in place that protect your system. For example, you may want to establish the routine to use screen savers to prevent damage to the monitor, or image "burn in," caused by the same image staying on the screen for a long time. Be cautious, though, that problems do not arise from screen savers interfering with other software applications on the network. Your hardware and software vendors can apprise you of known conflicts and help you to set up guidelines that will maximize your system's efficiency.

  Many instructions for the proper care of the computers will be specific to certain kinds of networks and software systems. Having plans before the network is up and running will prepare you for operational challenges that will occur in the future.

- ***Assign a responsible person.*** A person responsible for your network might attend Windows® training that will enable him or her to point out hazards to the rest of the staff, such as the danger of disks from home introducing viruses into the network. The goal is to create an atmosphere of open communication and develop dialogue between the staff and your implementation team.

- ***Offer Internet training.*** The Internet offers many sites for computer training, jargon, and definitions. This is a low-cost, timesaving method of enhancing your staff's knowledge base.

- ***Set up a demo.*** If available, set up a demonstration of your new software for your employees on a personal computer in your break room. Encourage staff to practice using the software and to become accustomed to it. Include members of the implementation team in your training sessions—they might be able to anticipate and eliminate problems before they occur.

- ***Secure advanced training.*** Beyond basic training that all employees will receive, key people should have further training, because maintaining a computer network and running software applications require many sophisticated skills. For example, many systems will automatically upload laboratory results into the electronic medical record, locating the appropriate patient chart based on name, social security number, birth date, or other identifier. If the software is not able to identify the appropriate chart, it often creates an error file that requires an appropriately trained person to go into the system, manually find the correct chart, and move the data. A staff member with computer training who can perform these kinds of tasks with a high degree of competency and accuracy is essential.

- ***Reward achievement.*** One way to increase employee morale during transition to EMR is to print achievement certificates for employees who have been through your training program. This helps to motivate and reward them for their effort in learning and setting up your new medical records system.

Developing Contingency Plans for System Failures

A medical practice using EMR must prepare for inevitable system failures due to circumstances such as power failure or system shutdown. When the user turns on the computer and gets a blank screen or an error message, there are many points in the system where the failure could have originated. If troubleshooting by your staff member in charge of the system is not able to immediately resolve the issue, it is important to have a backup plan. Training and precautions can prevent many problems and help to facilitate a quick resolution to those that happen.

Following are guidelines that will reduce the time your system is out of service and will enable you to keep seeing patients during down time.

- Keep handy a list of telephone numbers for all of your hardware and software vendors, help lines, and emergency numbers.

- Instruct employees to copy (by hand, if necessary) any error message that appears on their screen. This may help technical personnel solve the problem.

- Maintain a supply of backup paper forms and prescription pads for occasional down times.

- Develop a contingency plan for operating the office when the system is down. Information can be keyed into the computer later, when the system is up and running. Meanwhile, patients must still be seen, lab work done, and prescriptions written. One helpful precaution, for instance, is to print out the next day's schedule at the end of each day, or print the day's schedule first thing every morning.

- Be prepared for system failures by having a reliable external backup system in place to recover files. A number of solutions for system backup are available that vary widely in method and cost, including purchasing another network to "mirror" the primary network, tape backup systems that store tapes offsite (in case of fire or other catastrophe), and even Internet-based offsite backup. The appropriate choice for your practice will depend on the size and number of records your system stores.

Creating an Electronic Patient Population

The conversion of all of your patients' medical records from paper to electronic form may seem to be an impossible task, and would be quite difficult if it were necessary. However, since all charts in your practice do not belong to active patients, you may consider converting only records that show activity within the previous 13 months. Identify these patients from your billing records. This target group would capture all active patient files, as well as the records of patients who visit on an annual basis for routine physicals and examinations.

Generally, a minimal amount of information is necessary to create an electronic chart. Start with the following basics:

- Name

- Age

- Social Security Number

- Sex

When the patient arrives, the receptionist can enter additional information to complete the patient's record:

- Updated insurance information

- Addresses (home and work)

- Telephone numbers (home and work)

- Special notes, etc.

For some practices, creating electronic charts will be easy. Creating a patient population can occur in several ways, depending on the equipment and software you have.

- Using an interface software program, your staff can transfer information fields directly or indirectly from the current billing system to the new EMR.

- Without an interface, staff can sometimes manually download the information onto diskettes in a generic format (e.g., ASCII or comma-delimited text format) and then upload the data into your new EMR.

- If you do not have the capability to transfer the data, you must register each patient into the system manually. In this case, staff should input the information for the next day's patients each day.

Since editing electronic records is simple, the receptionist should ask all patients for any new or updated information at the beginning of each visit.

Maintaining Your Paper Charts

At this point, you will have a brand new electronic record that is empty of any relevant medical information, but your entire medical practice currently exists in paper charts, and for a time, you will still have to pull those charts. How should you effectively manage the transition from paper to computer?

Since patients' charts are legal medical records, you must maintain all of this information in some manner. Each state has separate laws governing these processes and procedures, so you should check with your state's governing boards for these regulations. In general, however, you must place all relevant paper-based medical information into the electronic medical record to care for your patients. When a patient comes in for a first electronic visit, the receptionist (or medical records person) should pull the paper chart and complete the computerized record as follows:

- All current medicines, allergies, and diagnoses can be transferred from the paper chart and entered into the EMR by a designated person (usually the physician).

- The physician can either dictate or fill out an electronic form to summarize the patient's care up to the implementation date of EMR.

- Using a highlighter, the physician then marks any pertinent lab values, EKG reports, and other data to manually enter into the EMR. Since physicians routinely summarize old medical records from other physicians, writing the transition should be equally uncomplicated.

  Surprisingly little information will be manually entered into the EMR. Most lab values will be normal and can be archived by recording only a few routine numbers. On a normal complete blood count (CBC), for example, the hemoglobin, hematocrit, platelets, and perhaps white blood count (WBC) might be recorded, with the rest of the values archived.

- The paper chart is then used as an archive for anything that cannot be placed into the EMR. EKG findings can be summarized into an EMR, but the EKG itself must be physically filed.

Updating and Reviewing Your System

After your new system is installed and operating, you and your staff will quickly settle into a new routine, part of which should be the review and updating of your system. Software and hardware developments aside, your staff should make a habit of looking for new and innovative ways to refine the care and service available in your office.

In a few years, your office will use dozens of different software programs, mostly integrated into a cohesive system for office automation. Medical office computer systems today typically come preloaded with word processor, spreadsheet, calendar, database, and Internet access (browser) software, along with programs to handle various other routine functions. The consumer is licensed to use the software he or she purchases as a part of the computer system. After the initial purchase, the licensee buys most software by subscriptions with updates and improvements a regular occurrence.

As a part of your ongoing maintenance and system review, make sure you and your staff do the following:

- *Stay involved with your vendors.* Regular contact with your vendors gives you the best chance to influence future upgrades, and staying abreast of scheduled releases will help you avoid future conflicts among the many providers you are likely to employ.

- *Keep a wish list.* One approach to influencing vendors is to keep an active "wish list" for your staff. As they write down glitches, suggested improvements, or desired new features, patterns might appear that can direct you to an underlying problem. Similar problems with two software programs, for instance, might suggest a questionable hardware component causing problems with both. These problems and subsequent solutions will only come to the forefront if you have a system in place to review routinely how you are using your office automation system.

- *Keep a support services list.* Keep a centralized list of all software support telephone and fax numbers, E-mail addresses, and vendor support staff personnel. When a problem occurs, immediately document it and contact the primary vendor whose product you think might be responsible. You might also consider making your other vendors aware of the problem by sending them a For-Your-Information memorandum. This will promote cooperation among vendors and foster a team approach to keeping your system updated.

- *Conduct periodic reviews.* Periodic reviews of how you are using your system are vital. Your vendors should be willing to come on-site and review your system's performance based on their knowledge of the product. These visits can also give you an opportunity to educate them about your particular office flow. An outside vendor's evaluation of your practice can give you a fresh, unbiased perspective to compare with your own internal review.

The process of switching from paper to electronic medical records is a complex and lengthy one that will be achieved more quickly and smoothly if appropriate groundwork has been laid. If you have carefully assessed your practice's needs and followed up with appropriate actions, your practice will be poised to make a successful move to EMR.

CHAPTER 3

Becoming Familiar with Computer Systems

Before moving a practice into the computer domain, the physician and practice manager are wise to attain a working knowledge of what makes up the electronic office. Much like the medical profession, the computer world uses its own specialized language. Becoming familiar with its basic terminology will prepare you to converse with vendors and give you confidence for making the best decisions. Along the way, you will learn a great deal about EMR and computerizing an office.

You do not need a degree in computer science to grasp this technology. Nevertheless, the exercise requires you to learn some new concepts and to acquire more than basic knowledge in order to make sound business decisions and get the most out of your system. Along the way, you may hear new terms and theories that you may not immediately understand; when this occurs, ask for further explanation until you are satisfied.

You (and your staff) really *do* need to understand computer systems to use them effectively. Although it may be tempting to believe that you can just plug a system in and have someone show you what to do, productive use of EMR requires that users develop a basic understanding of the system's components and architecture. Developing someone within your office who understands the system and how to work with it will be critical to your overall satisfaction with EMR, ensuring that you will have the technical support to stay up and running and the ability to customize the system to suit your own practice style.

Relational Databases

The cardinal concept behind EMR is the relational database. Simply defined, a *database* is the place where all of your data is stored (sometimes a database is described as a giant filing cabinet with millions of drawers). In a *relational* database, you have the ability to figuratively ask two or more drawers in the cabinet how they relate to each other, and they will open for you and tell you about their relationship without your searching through them.

In a medical relational database, every data element (e.g., subjective system, vital signs, objective physical exam finding, laboratory value, diagnoses, medication, treatment modality) occupies a unique field, and any fields can be linked. You can search, track, retrieve, and combine data to generate reports for use in your practice. In contrast, report generation from the paper record is nearly impossible because of the extensive time required to access and search records.

Most relational database software programs use Structured Query Language (SQL) in their programming. SQL programming incorporates specific formats and protocols to make it easier to locate information. Assume, for example, that you want to know which of your patients with diabetes have taken Drug X and whether this drug, if taken for more than a year, had a positive influence on their diabetes without inflaming their liver. If you were to review paper charts for this information, answering this question would require hundreds of hours of research to attain a statistically meaningful answer. Yet today, using SQL-based queries (questions phrased in a way computers can understand), you can ask and answer these kinds of questions with just a few keystrokes.

We, as physicians, must all become comfortable with asking more questions than in the past because now we can provide the answers. Using SQL queries with a relational database (e.g., your practice medical records) will enable heath care providers to analyze the practice of medicine in real time. For instance, when a new drug enters the market and is prescribed for tens of thousands of people, physicians will become aware of side effects and disease improvement parameters as they occur. Perhaps this knowledge will even precede the published results of multiple Phase Four studies that tell us how drugs react once they are released into the general population, since we will be tracking how they work while our patients are using them.

Hardware, Software, and Connectivity

The computer industry terms the physical components of a computer "hardware," a term that encompasses such devices as servers, terminals, networks, printers, alternative input devices, portable input devices, modems, etc. The following descriptions of hardware will be brief; we will illustrate applications of these components throughout the text. When you see an italicized word in the following definitions, it means you can find further information about the item later in this chapter or in the glossary at the end of this book.

Networks

"Network" means several different things in computer terminology. In this book, we use the term "network" to refer to two things:

- *Physical networks.* The *physical network* is the wiring that connects people to each other, either inter-office or intra-office. The physical network is the vehicle people use to exchange information, whether the distance between them is a matter of feet or miles.

  Speed on a network is very important. No matter how fast your *server* and your *terminal* are, if you have a slow network, you will spend long periods in front of a blank computer monitor. Waiting becomes annoying very quickly as you see productive time wasting away.

- *Conceptual networks.* The *conceptual network* is the state of people being on a network, for example, through the *Internet* or the connection among your own office staff. The conceptual network is the linking of different people at different places to share the same information, as in a user network.

LAN, WAN, and INTRANET are other networking terms you will hear when you are exploring your options for an EMR system. These are specific types of network designs (architectures) that differ from each other in a number of significant ways.

- A *LAN* is a local-area network in which local servers are generally hardwired to terminals in the same location. We would likely find these today in doctors' offices with one location and in small group practices. With a LAN, all network hardware is accessible on-site and therefore is easier to maintain and troubleshoot.

- A *WAN*, the next step up in complexity, is a wide-area network, usually linking two or more offices and/or locations over telephone lines. With a WAN, some or all terminals are in different locations than the server(s).

- An *INTRANET* can incorporate both LANs and WANs. An Intranet is a network that forms its own smaller version of the Internet. All the users can share and exchange information by accessing the main database. Medical groups with primary care and subspecialty doctors are using this very common model for referrals, authorizations, notes, and sharing different parts of the patient's medical chart.

Security, which we address later, becomes an issue with all networks and is a major consideration when we talk about patient information leaving the four walls of your office.

Servers

Although in years past the term "server" conjured the image of a massive piece of equipment sitting in a room by itself, today's server will look much like any other computer in your office. The pure definition of a server is "a computer that runs the main application(s) and/or stores centralized data." Servers are used only in offices that have *client-server* networks, which handle data processing centrally and offer access to the processed data through terminals that are networked together.

The server can be local or remote.

- *Local.* If your practice is self-contained in a single location, your computer system will likely be housed entirely within your office. In a local setting, your server will be in one room, and every terminal in your office will connect to that server through the network.

- *Remote.* If you have more than one location, if you want to have access from home or from the hospital, or if you are a part of a larger group, you will set up your server to operate from a remote setting.

In remote-server settings, economies of scale become important factors in purchasing decisions. The more money you can invest in a server for speed and storage capacity, the more efficient it will be. Economies of scale come into play as cost is spread among more users, allowing a lower per user cost.

A single-user EMR system is possible (since some single-user software exists), but even in a solo practice, this option is not popular because of efficiency and security problems. When a practice uses only one computer as both server and client, it is usually placed in an office by itself with access limited to designated users.

The server is the "brain" of the office. Although standard computers can be used as servers, the consumer often chooses to invest in a computer that has more speed and storage capacity, a higher capacity for add-on components, and other features. Two major contenders in the marketplace for moderate to large-sized systems are IBM and Hewlett-Packard. Prices currently begin at $5,000 for a bare-bones version; you can then customize and can go as high as tens of thousands of dollars.

All servers are very fast and can perform multitasking (carrying out more than one discrete operation at a time). With a standard computer, the computer can perform only one task while another user waits; in contrast, a multitasking server allows one user to access a patient's medication list while letting others simultaneously handle billings, print practice brochures, process E-mail, and use records to answer telephone queries.

One solution to the significant cost of a high-speed computer server with a large storage capacity is for two or more doctors to form a network and share the expense of the system. In this case, the investors choose a remote-access site to house the server and dedicate an employee to work with the information system and provide technological support. Depending upon the server chosen, up to 200–250 doctors may participate on one system.

Server Components

Most office networks in use today make use of "client-server architecture." In this kind of network, servers are complex, high-capacity computers that do most of the computing work for the office. Several different components make up a server.

- **Central processing unit (CPU).** Often called the "brain" of the computer, the CPU is the case and bones of the computer. When advertisements talk about type and speed of processor chip, they are referring to aspects of a CPU (an IBM-compatible Pentium® 266, for instance, is a CPU that uses a Pentium® chip and processes information at a speed of 266 megahertz). While these terms and numbers may at first seem difficult to understand, a good rule of thumb is to remember that the higher the number used to describe a CPU, the faster it will be. It is a good idea to purchase or lease the most advanced CPU available at the time you install your EMR system in order to ensure that the system will not become prematurely obsolete.

  The CPU does all the computing. In addition to a processor, it has random access memory (RAM), which determines the server's capacity to run all the applications that are open at one time. As with processor speed, the higher the number used to describe a CPU's RAM, the more powerful and fast the server will be.

- **Storage capacity.** A server also has one or more storage devices or disk drives. Hard drives, the most common kind of drive, are available in different sizes, and on servers are usually very large. *Disk drives* form the figurative filing cabinet rooms of your system.

  One term you may hear in discussion of disk drive storage capacity is "gigabyte." A gigabyte is a massive storage capacity—roughly equivalent to 700 standard floppy disks, which could hold 300,000 pages of plain text—that fits in a very small area. Hard disk drives are very compact and are getting smaller as technology advances. When considering storage drive capacity, you should base your choice on the number and size of patient files you will need for your practice, keeping in mind that advances in EMR software (e.g., the ability to store photos, movies, etc., in a patient record) may require more storage capacity. As of this writing, servers are available with hard drive capacities up to 9 gigabytes. Your hardware vendor should be able to guide you to appropriately-sized hard drives.

  Another data storage device you will hear about is the CD-ROM. With a CD-ROM drive, you can read CD-ROMs that store patient education material for use by both patients and office staff. Recently, the development of CD "burners" has offered another permanent record archiving option, since blank CDs may be purchased and loaded with data only once. CDs may eventually become a simple way to achieve permanent, archival backup of critical data.

- **Operating systems.** Another element of the server is the operating system, or platform. An operating system is basically the lowest level of language your server can understand, and all of the programs you run on your system must speak this same fundamental language.

  Names of some of the more popular operating systems are DOS, Windows®, UNIX, Macintosh, and OS2. Even within these operating systems, segmentation occurs, e.g., Windows® 95 in contrast with Windows® NT. Other technical deviations also occur among operating systems (for example, early versions of Windows® were not a true operating system, but a slightly higher-level language that "sat on top" of the DOS operating system). The operating system determines how applications will run on the system. Most importantly, the operating system and software you choose must be compatible. (A few programs can run cross-platform, but most are very specifically written for one operating system.)

  Network technology is rapidly advancing, with changes announced frequently. Before making a purchasing decision, you should investigate for which platform(s) the industry is creating software and factor this into your operating system selection decision. Good resources for researching this are the Internet, information technology magazines, and the information technology department within your health care system. Software vendors can also be good resources if you can steer discussion away from their specific products. When the time comes for evaluating EMR software, ask your prospective vendors to explain the operating system compatibilities and requirements of the software you are considering, and check out the information you receive with other sources to get a feel for where this product is in its level of development.

Terminals

Terminals, or "clients," are the main input devices in a networked computer system—your point of access to the medical record. The more terminals you have throughout the office, the better access will be. Every employee needs some access to the system at some point, whether through a terminal or a portable input device (see below) to make entries into the chart. Depending on how much processing power you need in each workstation, there may be several options when you are choosing terminals for your system.

How is it, you may wonder, that you can get complete documents from a library in Germany in a matter of seconds over the Internet, yet it takes three minutes for your hospital's computer system to generate an x-ray report? The difference lies in whose processor is used to perform major information processing tasks. When you are on the Internet, high-speed servers in a remote location (perhaps even another country) are retrieving the information you want, processing it, and sending the results to your computer screen through your modem, which connects your computer to other computers through telephone lines.

- **"Fat" clients.** Many existing client-server networks require the terminal to use its own processing power for all information processing functions, which means that the client machine must be memory-rich with a powerful processor. PCs of this sort can cost several thousands of dollars per unit. Also known as a "fat clients," these units can substantially increase the hardware costs of putting a network into a medical office. Until recently, most networks used fat clients, and servers stored data but did not usually manipulate them in any way.

- **"Thin" clients and "dumb" terminals.** The computer industry has recently introduced new technology that allows the use of a "thin client," or "dumb" terminal. With thin-client architecture, data manipulation is done on the server rather than the terminal.

  In the earlier Internet example, for instance, the essential processing power comes through a remote server on the Internet. Your personal computer (the client) is only receiving and displaying the information from this remote server. Nowadays, in fact, you do not really need the power of a PC to use the Internet; stripped-down "Internet-only" machines are on the market, as are devices used to access the Internet through your own television set. These options are much less expensive than powerful PCs and are good examples of "dumb" terminals.

  Since it is the server that runs the application in thin-client architecture, extreme speed and power are not necessarily vital at every workstation. Dumb terminals can allow staff access to information, but they will not be able to input changes or revisions to documents or records. Because of their lack of functionality, dumb terminals are relatively inexpensive, and using them for some office locations can save you money.

Portable Input Devices

Since you cannot carry a PC with you wherever you go, and since the space in your office limits the number of PCs you can set up permanently, using portable input devices is an obvious alternative. A portable device must be available for your use when you are in the office, at home, or in the hospital.

- **Laptop computers.** The most common portable input devices, laptops are small enough to carry home or to the hospital when you make rounds. One option for office use is to plug in your laptop when you are in the exam room. Since most of your patients are already familiar with laptops, they are not likely to find them intimidating.

- **Personal digital assistants.** Another category of tools available in the medical practice is personal digital assistants, or PDAs. These are small equipment installed with handwriting recognition programs. You can take notes and write down other information onto these assistants, then plug them into your system and transfer the data later. Some software companies are developing medical software designed to interface and integrate with your main computer system.

- **Dictation and transcription.** While this system is not new, it is currently the method that allows both the physician and the staff to make the transition to electronic medical records with the least amount of pain. If you currently use dictation and transcription, EMR will not change your practice drastically. If you do not currently dictate your notes, we encourage you to start. The more comfortable you are with dictation, the better you will be able to make the transition to EMR.

The last input option is for the physician to key in his or her notes directly. Unless the physician has attained a high level of speed and accuracy in keyboarding, however, this is the least efficient use of time.

Image Output Devices (Printers)

Every medical practice should have at least one high-quality laser printer in the office for creating hard copies of letters and printing prescriptions. Continuous-feed printers (trackfeed or formfeed printers that use paper with perforated, removable edges) are useful for printing jobs where quality is not an issue, as with large batches of billing. Special label printers are also sometimes useful for addressing appointment reminder postcards and other special-event notices (most professional-quality laser printers will also print labels; ask your hardware vendor about these capabilities).

In large offices, you may choose to set up your printers in zones or work groups so that several users access the same printers. In such a configuration, printers are zoned by common location and/or by similar tasks. As an example, the staff in billing and collections would use the same printers, and their software would automatically send their work to a designated printer by job type. When the billing clerk is preparing statements, then, the software will select and send the statement to the continuous-feed printer. When the same clerk writes a collection letter, however, the software sends the print job to the laser printer designated for correspondence.

Image Input Devices

Fresh, new information technology appears constantly in the light speed evolution of the computer industry. Since much information that is found on a medical chart is not easily entered by keyboard, we need other ways of transferring that information to the record. Innovations such as image input devices improve the speed of data entry and provide a way to get information into a computer without keying it in. Electronic scanners, digital cameras, and digital movies are three current means of getting hard data into the system.

- **Scanners.** Current technology allows for scanning, storage, and entry of images, such as x-rays and electrocardiograms, into an electronic medical record. (If the x-rays and EKGs are digitally produced, in fact, EMR software can store the original image without scanning. Most EKG machines currently on the market record results digitally and can easily transmit them anywhere, even to your EMR, if you have an interface built into your system. Any other office equipment that generates electronic information potentially can interface as well.)

  For documents that have not been stored digitally, the user may transform the data into digital form with a *desktop scanner* by feeding a flat document (either text or graphic) through the device. A digitized image of that document will then appear on the computer screen, and the user can either manipulate this image further (see *Text Recognition Devices*), or move it directly into the appropriate storage place in the chart, i.e., into the note section. Another device, convenient for larger or odd-sized documents, photographs, pictures, or bound documents, is the flatbed scanner. The flatbed scanner generally has a higher resolution than a desktop scanner. In recent years, scanners of both types have become very affordable and are a valuable addition to any office.

- **Digital cameras.** One obvious use for a digital camera in the medical practice is to take photographs of patients. Having a picture of the patient in the medical record improves security and enhances patient service. If you have 10,000 patients, and you are not sure with whom you are speaking over the telephone, a photograph in the chart allows you to jog your memory, and when you recognize the patient, prior encounters will come to mind that may help you evaluate the situation. The camera may also be used to document locations and/or severity of injuries or external symptoms.

- *Digital movies.* Another of the impressive image input devices available on the market, digital movie cameras are especially useful for specialties such as cardiology, where EKGs are filmed and stored. Another possible application is documenting physical injuries and recording what the patient is able to do. Digital movies would serve well for substantiating your patients' workers' compensation claims, motor vehicular accident-related injuries, and other disabilities.

  One current drawback with digital movies, however, is their requirement for massive amounts of storage space on the server's hard drive(s). As digital movie storage formats and compression technologies improve, it is possible that movies may become common parts of a medical record.

Developers are constantly making advances in digital image input technology, and manufacturers are refining products available in the marketplace. Watch for these products to improve and be ready to take advantage of the benefits they will bring to your practice.

Text Recognition Software

A scanned piece of paper containing text can be stored in a computer in two ways. One way is to save the text in as an "image," but this method takes up a great deal of disk storage space compared to storing only the text itself. Data from text stored as images also cannot be placed into a relational database, and therefore are not useful for EMR. This means that if a lab result from five years ago was saved as an image, a current user cannot search and retrieve that data and place it into a report. This is a drawback that only manually reentering the data can remedy. For most practices, this solution is too time-prohibitive.

A better way to handle scanned text is to have the computer "read" the words and then store the data as a text document. The software that makes this process possible, called Optical Character Recognition (OCR) software, allows storage and retrieval of data in a relational database and eliminates the problem of reentering data.

Optical Character Recognition software is available on the market and evolving rapidly. Many EMR packages incorporate this feature as part of their system. Once the users convert a document to digital text, they can then use it in the database. At this time, however, the error rate is relatively high, especially when scanning documents generated with serif fonts. (Serifs are extra curls, crosses, and curves that give the type some flair; to see the difference yourself, compare Times New Roman, a serif font, to Arial, a sans-serif font.) If a physician is scanning a document from which he or she must make medical judgments (for which he or she is legally responsible) into a database, he or she requires an error rate near zero. Therefore, OCR must be used with a great deal of caution, and the accuracy of scanned text must be checked thoroughly.

Voice Recognition Technology

Would you find it enjoyable to talk to a machine and see your words printed instantaneously? The concept of voice-to-text sounds appealing, but this medium is not yet ready for practical application.

Extensive research and development in this area have occupied software companies for the last few years, but much work remains to be done. Although some programs on the market actually work, these instruments still tend not to recognize a person's voice consistently, and most require a slow, careful pronunciation called discrete speech. Put simply, when using this technology, you . . . need . . . to . . . space . . . between . . . each . . . word . . .comma . . . and. . .tell. . . the. . .program. . .exactly. . .what. . . to. . .type. . .period. If one does not speak slowly and distinctly, the error rate increases dramatically. And to compensate for the deficiencies in the program, the physician must edit his or her notes while dictation is in progress. The time you spend correcting your text makes it prohibitive for most users. To remedy these problems, software developers are working hard on continuous (or "normal") speech recognition programs, but these are not yet fully functional.

The present imperfections in the continuous voice speech technology (error rate and lack of speed) make this option currently unfeasible for use in most medical practices. Voice recognition software does, however, learn from its mistakes and gets better the more you use it, making it somewhat more useful for repetitive entry like radiology reports. In a diverse practice such as family medicine, however, the plethora of dictation reduces the practicality of voice recognition software.

Evaluating whether this technology is appropriate for your practice requires three considerations: (1) a detailed knowledge of what you wish to dictate, (2) awareness of how patient you will be with the software, and (3) the error rate of the software. When the technology's limitations are acceptable to the end user, and when the products demonstrate an approved cost/benefit ratio, voice recognition may finally become more than a fancy and frustrating toy.

Harwired Deliveries, Infrared Transmissions, or Radio Frequency Broadcasts

The industry continues to debate the best way to get portable devices to work effectively on a network. Three communication options are available: hardwired delivery, infrared transmission, and radio frequency broadcasting.

- *Hardwiring* computers together is an expensive and disorderly project. Unless you have the luxury of building new office space, adding a hardwired electronic medical records network to your office will involve moving furniture and equipment, cutting holes in walls, and having workers climb through your ceilings. One way to reduce the chaos of network installation is to use wireless technology.

- *Infrared* transmission works like familiar household remote controls, allowing your network to be wireless, but it does require a direct line of sight to a receiver. Therefore, you must place a receiver that is hardwired to the server in each room. Infrared transmission is a popular option for networking today.

- *Radio frequency* broadcasting is considered the best option of the three, according to current consensus. Radio frequency is a high-powered broadcasting device that has great range, goes through walls (eliminating the need for hardwired relay sensors), and is very fast. One advantage of radio frequency broadcasting is that it updates about every thirty seconds. This means that if someone in your office makes a change to a record, or if you change a record and you want to go back and look at it, you can get as close as thirty seconds to "real time." Usually, installing only one or two transmitters throughout your office is sufficient to have an effective system. This technology also allows for easier expansion into future areas of your clinic; therefore, the entire network does not require up-front planning.

Backup Strategies

Perhaps the most important part of your practice's new computer system after the server is the combination of equipment and software that form your backup system. Electronic storage of patient charts and other sensitive, confidential information demands that ultimate care be taken to protect and preserve the data from numerous threats. Among the things that can damage or destroy your data files are hardware failures, software glitches, power outages, theft, employee sabotage, human error, and natural disasters like fires and floods.

Once you have implemented EMR, your practice will exist primarily as information. Backing up your data on a regular basis will be the most important way to protect your practice from unforeseen dangers. Ask your vendors, especially, for their recommendations about backup systems.

When evaluating backup strategies, keep in mind that a backup system must meet several important needs:

- *Capacity.* The backup system(s) you choose must have enough storage space to copy not only all your data files but also all your programs. This means that it must be able to hold at least as much information as the space you are using on your server. If it can hold all this information on just one piece of storage media (tapes, disks, etc.), all the better.

- *Expandability.* As your practice grows and technology allows you to easily store more graphic and textual information about your patients, you will need more backup space. The system(s) you choose must be able to grow to meet these added demands.

- *Ease of use.* No matter how important backup is, staff will be reluctant to do it if it is time-consuming and tedious. The easier and more automated a system is, the more likely it is that your critical data will be available the morning after a disaster. Backup systems that require no human involvement whatsoever, such as overnight archiving using special software, or Internet archiving, are probably the best insurance that your backup will be performed regularly.

- *Reliability.* Backup systems are useless if they are prone to break down. Years ago, for instance, people backed up their computer data on floppy disks. On occasion, however, the floppy disks themselves became unstable or corrupted, and data that was supposed to be backed up disappeared in computer crashes. In the past few years, backup media and methods have increased the reliability of data backup dramatically.

  Another reliability consideration is the geographic location of data. If data are simply backed up from one part of a server to another, for instance, there is very little protection against a disaster that destroys the entire server (theft, flood, or fire, for instance). Because of this consideration, more people are backing up their files off-site in recent years than ever before. Better still, some are backing up data both locally and off-site, since the odds that a disaster will concurrently destroy data at both places are astronomically low.

Most backup systems today are designed around one or more of the following strategies. Investigate and weigh the costs and potential benefits of these systems, and keep in mind the impact that losing all of your patient records would have on your practice.

- *Additional stationary hard drives.* One of the simplest methods of data backup is to install a second hard drive on your server or PC and use a software program to copy the data from one hard drive to another on a regular basis. This method, of course, does not safeguard against physical destruction of the computer, and it also leaves you (or your staff) with the temptation to store additional data on the second hard drive when the first fills up. Although this is a low-cost option, it leaves some important reliability issues unaddressed.

- *Removable hard drives.* Your hardware vendors are able to use special kits to install a slot on the front of your computer into which you can slide removable hard drives. Using three or four hard drives on a rotating basis, you can then store the drive not currently in use in a different office or building, thereby safeguarding data separately from the physical computer. The drawback with this system, however, is that someone must physically perform the backup function each day and transport the hard drives to their remote storage location. This increases the likelihood that backup will not be done regularly.

- *Tape drives.* A very popular method of backup on many systems, tape drives are magnetic storage devices that are usually (but not always) separate from the CPU. They offer many of the same advantages and disadvantages as hard drive backup systems. Also, they must access data sequentially, which means that if the data for which you are searching was stored 7/8 of the way through the backup process, the tape drive will need to physically "fast forward" the tape that far to reach it. Often tape drives are used to back up entire systems, including programs, rather than just data files.

- *CD-ROM archiving.* With the advent of affordable "CD burners," it is possible to go a step beyond backup and actually archive digital information for permanent storage in a very small area. CDs can be used, for instance, to hold several patients' scanned paper records, like EKGs and other graphic test results. The CDs may then be numbered and referenced in the electronic medical record for quick and easy location of these records. Because CDs cannot be rewritten, however, they are not a practical everyday backup alternative.

- *Internet archiving.* With the rapid growth of Internet-based enterprises and the growing popularity of permanent network connections to the Internet, it is now possible to back up your data to a remote location without thought or effort. By signing up with an Internet backup service, you ensure that your data will be accessed and backed up according to your specifications and stored remotely (often from another state). While some people may have concerns about the confidentiality issues involved in Internet backup, encryption and compression of data do make this a secure option.

Whichever backup method(s) you eventually choose to employ, it is important that you have a strong backup system in place before you create even one record in EMR. Use your backup system faithfully and you will be safeguarded against almost all forms of long-term data loss.

Final Thoughts on Purchasing Hardware

The options and choices you will be facing when you research your new system may at times threaten to become overwhelming, but don't despair. You will learn a good deal from vendors and, as you move forward, will also develop a good instinct for identifying those system components that will meet your needs. Do not feel the need to rush through the selection process; evaluate each network component calmly and thoroughly, and be sure to keep asking vendors questions if you feel you don't completely understand what they are offering. With common sense and persistence, you will find that building a system to meet your needs is much less daunting than you may initially have suspected.

Once you have your hardware in place, it will be time to evaluate EMR software. The next chapter walks you through the decision-making process step by step.

CHAPTER 4

Evaluating EMR Software

Now that you have learned the why's and the how's of moving to an electronic medical records software environment, you can consider specific software products. All vendors will use attractive graphics and fast, efficient demonstrations to impress you. Before you schedule the first demonstration with a vendor, you need to prepare yourself to evaluate the EMR properly. In this chapter, we will teach you to assess products from a technical standpoint.

Begin your assessments using the following approach:

- Be aware that EMR software is task-specific.

- Thoroughly review your office workflow first to gain a detailed knowledge of the individual tasks performed in your office.

- Understand your problems and operational goals.

- Rely on your office manager to be an integral part of the EMR evaluation and selection team.

- Spend time with your front office personnel and clinical staff, particularly your nurse, to gain insight into what they do and greatly improve your ability to evaluate the EMR product properly.

- Keep in mind that the physician, for whom time equals productivity, is the end-user.

Core Vendor Software versus Best-of-Breed Software

A fundamental question to answer about office automation is how much support and software you want each vendor to supply. Two basic strategies, at opposite ends of the spectrum, are possible choices, but each organization's approach will likely fall somewhere between the two extremes.

- **Core vendor software.** At this end of the spectrum, you will have a single vendor who will meet all of the needs and functions for your office or health care system, including EMR, billing, scheduling, managed care, laboratory, and home health functions (among others), each specifically adapted to your operation. The core vendor approach integrates remote communication, central versus local repositories of data, and all of the other complexities of office automation into one software package.

  The core vendor approach offers several advantages. Working with only one vendor streamlines communication and reduces the need for multiple phone calls to handle problems. Vendors who offer core services often obtain volume discounts from manufacturers that you would not be able to get individually. It is also easier for staff members who administer the network to plan for your needs, since they will handle only one brand of software.

Having a single vendor can also simplify forecasting of capital investment and expenses by permitting you to attain one price for all you will be purchasing. Usually, no expensive interface software is necessary to communicate among disparate software packages in a single-vendor system.

A one-package-does-everything strategy has several disadvantages, however. If you have one supplier for all your automation needs, and you decide to make a change, you may need to alter your entire computer system rather than just a part of it.

Another disadvantage to the core vendor solution is the rapid obsolescence and evolution of technology. Programmers writing software programs and developers of computer systems achieve major technologic leaps in very short periods of time. It is possible that by the time a software company's programmers complete the development of a comprehensive software package, its platform may be outmoded (for example, a new scheduling system written specifically for Windows® 95 is released at the same time as Windows® 98).

A company that specializes in one area of automation, such as billing software, will try to have the best billing software available. A specialty company will bring to bear a certain level of expertise when compared with a company trying to address all aspects of automation. Therefore, although a single software package may provide for all your needs, it will probably not represent the best-of-breed in each field.

■ **Best-of-breed software.** With the best-of-breed approach to office automation, the consumer uses multiple software packages and vendors and integrates the different components into an information system.

The multiple-component strategy offers many advantages over the core vendor system. First, most offices and health care systems have already attained some level of automation, usually for billing and practice management functions. These users save money, time, and effort if they can integrate their existing systems into the overall automation stratagem.

The best-of-breed approach also stimulates inherent competition among your vendors. Your electronic medical records software provider, for instance, will know that you can discard his software and purchase another if it fails to satisfy your needs and may therefore work harder to please you. The innate competition between vendors in the marketplace also provides you an opportunity to negotiate for better prices.

In addition, the best-of-breed software selection method allows you to upgrade individual areas of automation without disrupting other effective programs.

Best-of-breed technology also offers the benefit of having access to multiple providers of expertise. All of your vendors will try to solve technical problems, upgrade systems, and remain competitive in their respective markets. With multiple vendor relationships, you can benefit from their work and be assured that your computer system will remain at the forefront of technology.

The disadvantages to the multiple-vendor/software setup primarily center on lack of organization and communication. Programs need to communicate efficiently with one another, and since problem-solving is apt to require a team approach, your vendors must make sure this process is smooth for you.

A physician must know that expertise is available to keep the system running. Expertise will come from your staff, your health care organization, and your hardware, networking, and communications software vendors. This multiple-vendor/software approach demands a broader knowledge about computer systems than a single-vendor approach, because operational responsibilities are dispersed. One common problem is having two vendors blame each other for a problem, with neither ultimately providing a solution.

The best-of-breed approach largely uses interface engines, which combine computer hardware, software, and expertise to make two seemingly disparate computer systems communicate together. When your office enters a secondary insurance company's telephone number into a patient's chart, interface engines will allow the number to flow through the billing software, lab software, etc., and consistently land in the same place in each database.

From a technical standpoint, interfacing requires having an individual with a comprehensive knowledge of the systems adapt the hardware and software to ensure correct and dependable transfer of information. It also requires the cooperation of all vendors involved. These vendors must be willing to share their technical expertise with people outside their own companies.

Many health care systems are getting together with outpatient practices to standardize their applications and agree on certain parameters for their hardware and software tools. This cooperation will continue to evolve in coming years among providers. Keep track of the progress made in this area before choosing or updating your computer system by attending meetings concerning health care information systems and working directly with key administrators. A good place to start your education in IS technologies is the information systems director at your health system. He or she can give you an overview of the system in your medical community and will, in turn, educate you regarding the principles of the industry at large.

General Features of Electronic Medical Records

When viewing an EMR program for the first time, several features might quickly determine whether you wish to take an involved look at a particular product. A good way to test the usability of an EMR program is to try out a fully functional EMR demonstration program without instruction—a hands-on demonstration (if the distributor does not have a good demo, eliminate the program from your consideration). If you can maneuver around a demo intuitively, using only your reasoning and the information on the screen, you probably are viewing a good product.

The usability test is especially helpful if you are not very familiar with computers. If a less experienced person can maneuver around the software, staff will probably learn it easily, too. Software developers build most programs essentially the same way, and a practiced user becomes proficient at using software without much instruction.

Look for the following features during your own hands-on demonstration:

- The program should offer an easy-to-read summary screen for each patient so that you can quickly review the chart.

- Moving around the chart should be quick and simple. You should have the option of using either keystrokes or a mouse.

- Count the number of keystrokes necessary to use the product. Look with favor on those that require the fewest combinations.

- Look for consistencies within the program. If pressing the F1 key brings up a help screen, for instance (as it frequently does), it should do so throughout the entire program. If F1 has different functions in different areas of the EMR, the program is probably not very well designed.

- In the average business environment, speed of screen changes and updating of information is not a critical issue. In the practice of medicine, however, if you lose one minute per patient waiting for the computer to access information, you can easily waste enough time throughout the day to see two to three patients. Computer speed depends on several factors, including your file server, network, individual personal computer capabilities, number of users on the network, and software. When exploring your purchase options, question vendors closely regarding the efficiency of their software in a variety of settings.

- Most of the common functions of the EMR should be apparent. The program should *highlight* important information in some manner; often, programs prompt allowable functions by highlighting a bar or button on the screen.

- Select a program that automatically checks for drug-drug interactions and warns of drug allergies and reactions in an obvious way.

- EMR software should allow the user to create customized forms, notes, and so on. It should be sufficiently user-friendly that ordinary users can generate letters and documents as standard functions, not special features, of the software. The system should also permit instantaneous changes to user-defined features.

- The software you choose should facilitate diagnosis and procedure coding.

Selecting the Vendor

Selecting the vendor and the software are similar processes. Follow these steps:

- Identify the specific needs of your practice.

- Budget for a computer system, including initial purchase and yearly upkeep.

- Establish a schedule for research, purchase, installation, and implementation.

- Generate a request for proposal (RFP) based on above criteria in which you spell out the requirements and features you desire in a system and invite vendors to tell you about their products. A sample RFP follows for your reference.

Date

Mr. John Salesman
EMR Company
Address
City, State, Zip

Re: Request for Proposal for Purchase of Electronic Medical Records Software

Dear John:

Following is request for proposal for All About Care, L.P.C.'s, electronic medical records purchase. Please review the information carefully and submit a bid. All About Care is a family medical practice with a staff of four primary care physicians. The practice's primary location is 1001 Medical Center Drive, Center, State, with satellite offices at 2002 Get Well Lane and 3003 Feeling Better Way. The proposal should be for all three locations, with the understanding that other locations may be added in the future.

Practice styles vary among the physicians. Some doctors dictate and others write their documentation to the medical record. AAC requires a medical record system that accommodates users who have differing levels of computer knowledge, varied computer skills, and assorted work styles.

Scope of Service

An EMR system will be provided to each office to be used for both clinical and administrative functions of the medical practice. Key features include (but are not limited to) the following:

- integration with practice management software

- Web-based network connectivity

- integration with telemedical systems

- integration with workflow protocols

- integration with decision support

- maximum security levels to ensure confidentiality

- uses SNOMED™ and CPT™ for data encoding

- produces HEDIS or other performance measurement reports

The vendor will provide a list and prices for all necessary hardware and computer peripherals required for running the software. The vendor will work with the practice administrator to coordinate installation of all equipment.

Exhibit 4–1 continued...

Before selection of a system, we ask the vendor to provide a demonstration unit for use by employees. Once the purchasing decision is made, we request that the vendor present a time line for installation. Following installation, we ask that the vendor provide the practice staff on-site training.

After the initial stages are complete, the vendor will provide ongoing maintenance of the program. Occasionally, when new physicians join the practice, the vendor will be asked to work with the physician on individual training.

Quotation Deadline

Proposals are requested by December 31, 1998. If no response has been received by that date, your company will be eliminated from consideration. Please provide pricing both for cash payment and financing arrangements.

If you have any questions or need clarification on any of the above, please contact me at (800) 438-9673. Our fax number is (949) 345-5859.

Sincerely,

Gail Goodjob
Practice Administrator

Exhibit 4–1 continued...

Request for Proposal to Purchase an Electronic Medical Record System for an Ambulatory Setting

Introduction

ABC Family Care Center, LLC, founded in 1993, is a privately owned physician group of three physicians providing family health care services to the local service area. ABC Family Care Center will be selecting a vendor to supply an ambulatory electronic medical record system. This document serves as a Request for Proposal for vendors who wish to be considered during the selection phase.

Objectives

The overall objective is to evaluate and select an integrated Physician Practice Management System, Managed Care Administration System, and Electronic Ambulatory Medical Record System that will provide the following:

- The support necessary for high-quality, patient-focused care that is offered at a reasonable cost

- Real-time access to comprehensive patient and clinical information, immediate intervention based on established patterns of care, and better communications between patients and interdisciplinary providers

- The competitive advantage necessary to succeed in a managed care reimbursement environment

- Integration capabilities with a regional health information network for the purpose of data sharing

- Coding compliance for Medicare and other payers

Volume Assumptions

For the purpose of hardware and software configurations, vendors should use the following assumptions.

- Three-physician group

- Hardware and software resident in the group offices

- Practice Statistics

    Number of patients...4,000–5,000

    Number of visits...12,000

    Planned number of EAMR users 6

    Planned number of practice management users 3

    Planned number of workstations...16

Exhibit 4–1 continued...

Scope of the Request for Proposal

ABC is requesting information for a comprehensive Physician Practice Management System (with managed care function and Electronic Ambulatory Medical Record System) that includes the application areas listed below. ABC's primary approach is to have any vendor responding to the RFP to do so as a "prime vendor." ABC would prefer to accept proposals from firms who are willing to "subcontract" those portions of the integrated solution they cannot provide themselves. ABC will consider, as an alternative option, a "best of breed" approach to meet functional requirements and integration needs. *Submitters should be very specific in the introduction of their response as to the approach they have taken in the proposal.*

I. Physician Practice Management Functionality
    A. Appointment Scheduling
    B. Patient Registration
    C. Billing and Accounts Receivable
    D. Chart Tracking
    E. Eligibility/Benefits
    F. Referral Authorization management
    G. Claims Management
    H. Capitation Calculation/Risk Pool Management
    I. Provider Maintenance
    J. Patient Services Management
    K. Utilization Management/Reporting

II. Electronic Ambulatory Medical Record Functionality
    L. General System Characteristics
    M. Patient Clinical Information
    N. Patient Care Management
    O. Administrative
    P. Billing Data Requirements
    Q. Business Management/Reporting

III. General Requirements
    R. Electronic Data Interchange
    S. Report Writer
    T. Year 2000 Compliant

Exhibit 4–1 continued...

Definitions

The term "Vendor" shall mean a manufacturer or seller of products and/or services.

The term "Submitter" shall mean a Vendor that is submitting a response for consideration by ABC pursuant to this RFP.

The term "Contractor" shall mean a Vendor that enters into a binding contract agreement with ABC.

The "Finalist Vendor(s)" shall mean those Submitters selected to enter into the evaluation phase of the project.

Response Requirements

General Instructions

Please include a written point-by-point response to the functions listed above and your product's ability to meet these criteria. Each response must be cross-referenced to the correspondingly numbered item in the list above, describing in as much detail as possible your product's ability to meet this specification. All points must be addressed. Omissions may be grounds for rejection of your proposal.

ABC Contacts

Please direct any questions you may have to _____ at the number below. Your written response should be sent to:

> ABC Family Care Center, LLC
> Attn: _____
> 123 Main Street, Suite 321
> Anytown, USA 12345-5678
> 309 555 1212

Submittal

Each submittal shall be presented in a three-ring, loose-leaf binder. The complete response to the RFP shall include:

- A comprehensive point-by-point response to all items listed in the Scope of the Request for Proposal as outlined above

- An itemized list of exceptions (if any are taken)

- A list of five references

ABC is seeking information that meets the requirements as outlined. If more than one method of meeting these requirements is proposed, each shall be labeled and presented separately.

Exhibit 4–1 continued...

Submittal Deadline

ABC Family Care Center will receive and accept submissions until January 31, 1999, at 5:00 P.M., EST.

Teaming

Teaming between manufacturers and/or resellers (or value-added resellers offering service/ maintenance options) is permitted. However, in the Submittal response, the Submitter must specify all teaming partners/subcontractors by company name, contact person, and address.

The Contractor will be responsible for the performance of all teaming/partnerships.

Purchase orders and payments will be issued to the Contractor or designated team partner, and it will be their responsibility to issue purchase orders, schedule services, and pay all partners/ subcontractors directly. The manufacturer shall be responsible for all obligations regardless of which entity performs under any purchase order.

Pricing

The Submitter's response shall include specific, itemized pricing information on every aspect of purchasing an EMR System as described within this document, including but not limited to items of software, hardware, installation (including wiring), and maintenance agreements.

The Submitter will notify ABC of any pricing changes that occur during the evaluation process.

Evaluation Process

ABC will select two finalists from the written responses submitted for review, based on its evaluation of the proposals. Each Finalist Vendor must agree, upon request, to provide ABC scenario-based demonstrations of its EMR application solution and provide a list of appropriate sites where its EMR application solution is currently being used. The Vendor will be responsible for installing and uninstalling the EMR application solution.

The demonstration period is anticipated to begin March 1, 1999, and last approximately two weeks.

The site visits are anticipated to begin mid-March 1999, and last approximately two weeks.

- The criteria for evaluation are:

- The soundness of the respondent's approach

- The respondent's demonstrated competence and experience

- The qualifications and experience of the team members proposed to conduct the services offered

- Respondent's experience performing the requested services for other medical practices of various sizes

Exhibit 4–1 continued...

- The up-front and five-year-overall cost of goods and services to be provided for ABC's EMR solution

- The quality of references from past customers of respondent

- Respondent's demonstrated capability and financial resources to perform the work in the time projected

- Respondent's response to Technical and Functional Requirements

- Respondent's response to RFP

- Respondent's acceptance of pilot

Confidentiality

ABC will take reasonable precautions to ensure that the Submittals are held in confidence, provided, however, each Submitter agrees, by replying to this RFP, that ABC shall have no obligation of confidentiality and shall incur no liability for disclosure of information which

- Is in the public domain at time of disclosure

- Becomes publicly known through no wrongful act of ABC

- Is known or becomes known to ABC through disclosure by lawful sources other than the information

- Is disclosed by ABC pursuant to the requirement of governmental agency or any law requiring disclosure thereof.

ABC reserves the right to reject any or all submittals received. Non-acceptance of a submittal shall mean that another submittal was deemed more advantageous to ABC, or that all submittals were rejected. Submitters whose submittals were not accepted shall be notified after a binding contractual agreement between ABC and the successful Submitter exists or after ABC has rejected all submittals.

A Submitter shall promptly notify ABC of any ambiguity, inconsistency, or error that they may discover upon examination of the submittal documents.

Agreement

The award of a contract will not be based only on the lowest price. ABC will determine, at its sole discretion, which information best fulfills or exceeds the requirements of the RFP and is deemed to be in the best interest of ABC.

ABC reserves the right to negotiate, prior to an award, any contract that may result from this RFP.

Using Outside Resources

Computer and software vendors are understandably biased. They are prone to employ sales associates who may be too optimistic about the capabilities of their products. In reality, they may promise results that their software cannot achieve. Often an independent computer consultant can be helpful in assessing your needs and aiding in the development of your RFP. Other physicians who have advanced computer systems and electronic medical records applications in their practices serve as good resources as well, particularly if they have attained a high level of expertise and market exposure.

The purchase of software products warrants a healthy dose of skepticism by the purchaser. Be generous with the number of RFPs you send out, realizing that many proposals may not meet your needs. Narrow your field to the four or five best companies, and set up live, hands-on demonstrations. This will be your opportunity to find out how well the system fits in with your daily office routine.

Evaluating Vendors

Evaluate vendors along with software to be sure you can work successfully with them to achieve positive results.

- Organize your evaluation process using forms you have prepared before meeting with the vendors. Use a separate form for each vendor, asking specific questions of each. (See *Vendor Evaluation Form* on page 61)

- Find out what service and maintenance is available and what the charges are. Look over a maintenance agreement; find out whether training material is provided for an extra charge.

- Quality training and support for the purchased product are essential. Carefully evaluate the training and support policies of each prospective vendor and develop a definite plan with specifics regarding the number of trainers, time and equipment required, and so on. Obtain information about the product and training process through interviews or visits with the vendor's current clients. Ask your vendor whether there will be training personnel on-site during the first day or so of actual product use.

- From the information you obtain, assess how each vendor fits into the overall scheme, not just the capabilities of their product. Following is a list of questions you might ask when evaluating a product and its vendor. These questions do not directly address the capabilities of the company's EMR product. However, the answers should give you an idea of the vendor's position compared with your vision of your future and that of the health care industry. A company's philosophy is as sometimes as important as the specific features of its software.

Exhibit 4–2 **Vendor Evaluation Form**

Company Name: _____

Sales Associate: _____

Local Address: _____

    Street/Suite: _____

    City: _____ State: _____ Zip Code: _____

Telephone Number: _____ Fax Number: _____

E-mail Address: _____

Web Site: _____

Home Office/Regional Office Address: _____

    Street/Suite: _____

    City: _____ State: _____ Zip Code: _____

Number of years in business: _____

How many offices currently use the product?_____
(Obtain a complete list, not a referral list, of practices that have this product running in their offices.)

How much demographic information does your EMR hold? _____

Will this product communicate with our billing system?_____

Will this product communicate with our lab system? _____

What other interfaces exist today and with what other products? _____

What interfaces are planned currently? _____

Are your engineers willing to work closely with other companies? _____

Who specifically handles software support?_____

Who will help with network problems? _____

What kind of server terminal do we need to run the program? Operating System?_____

    Megahertz? _____ RAM? _____

    Processor?_____ Network? _____

What will your product require in future hardware and network upgrades? _____

_____

_____

_____

Exhibit 4–1 continued...

How will this software handle special information I need to put into the EMR to track/study patients?

_____

_____

_____

What are your plans and capabilities for remote access? _____

_____

_____

_____

What are your plans and capabilities for central repositories? _____

_____

_____

_____

What are the EMR product capabilities (use a separate sheet to make notes during the demo)? _____

_____

_____

_____

Selecting the Software Program

The key to success in all aspects of office automation, particularly electronic patient records, is people. The electronic medical record must deliver benefits to physicians, clinical staff, health care managers, payers, and, most important, patients. Look for and rate the following features in the software systems you consider purchasing.

- *How does this program automate workflow?* The EMR must automate the entire workflow, not just the patient encounter, and not just the chart. The workings of a medical practice include tasks like scheduling, ongoing projects, receiving and delivering messages, preparation of reports and documents, and more. In a paper system, messages are attached to various items in patient charts, usually by paper clips or stick-on notes. *Will this system automate these functions in your daily practice operations?*

- *Will the software allow multiple users access to the same file?* One of the greatest advantages of the computerized medical record is concurrent functionality. When providers break the "one user at a time" stranglehold imposed by paper charts, they work more efficiently. This feature allows the implementation of a true teamwork model for the encounter, because several team members can both view and enter data about the same encounter from different workstations without interference. *Does this system allow access to more than one user at a time?*

- *Is the software "Year 2000 (Y2K) Compliant"?* You should insist on a product that will handle the change in millenium without requiring you to purchase any additional software. Better yet, the system you purchase should already be written so that it will know that "00" means "2000," not "1900." Do not settle for a product from a vendor who has not yet addressed or resolved this critical issue.

- *Does the program allow immediate access to clinical data?* A computerized medical record system must be able to find and display a chart quickly. *Does the program allow the clinician to see data within the chart in new useful ways not possible with paper? Can the user gain more information to arrive at competent conclusions?*

- *Does the system accommodate different styles of data entry?* There must be a flexible choice of data entry methods to satisfy needs that differ widely, depending upon whether physicians are primary care or specialist, office- or hospital-based, young or old, computer-literate or technophobic. The *gradual adoption* of template-based data entry methods, using a mouse or pen to select options, will take place in areas where it is appropriate. (As we have previously explored, new technologies for human-computer interaction like voice and handwriting recognition are moving along in development but have not yet proved practical in daily use.) *What are the various means of data entry offered by this software program?*

- *Does the system offer clinical decision support, i.e., preventive care reminders, medications, allergies, correct dosing, and contraindications?* To be most effective, clinical decision support should be delivered at the moment of decision-making. Preventive care reminders enhance compliance with immunization and screening guidelines, and other decision support focuses on particular, risk-prone aspects of care. In most EMR packages, as more clinical information becomes available within the record, higher levels of decision support become available. *How well does the system you are considering offer clinical decision support?*

- *Does this system's structure and coding allow measurement of quality and outcomes?* As a result of work by standards committees, research by informatics groups, and increased awareness of the necessity of computerizing patient records, several products now offer coding and structure features that enable you to measure care quality and outcomes.

  Several products now offer SNOMED™ (Systematized Nomenclature of Medicine) coding as supplements to the ICD coding of diagnoses. In addition, the LOINC (Logical Observation Identifier Names and Codes) encoding standard for laboratory test results allows EMR systems to organize them into flowsheets and graphs without requiring the time-consuming construction of individual mappings from each laboratory's test numbering system. SNOMED and LOINC do not replace ICD and CPT coding; they complement them. *Does the program you are considering support several coding systems?*

- *Does this system identify who "owns" the data?* Health systems with a network of providers using EMR must know whose information they are using. For example, if a primary care physician (PCP) uses data that a referral specialist enters after seeing the PCP's patient, the PCP must be able to validate that test results and notes came from the specialist. Systems must be designed so that data aligns with the realities of business and data ownership. *Does the system make such identification quick and easy?*

- *Is the system designed to become HIPAA (Health Insurance Portability and Accountability Act of 1996) compliant?* Briefly, with this legislation, Congress declared that a set of universal standards should be devised and implemented for all electronic transactions within

American health care system. Once the standards are determined, the law will require compliance within 24 months.

The standards mandated by HIPAA will govern electronic interchanges of claims information, enrollment and disenrollment in health plans, first reports of injury, and referral certifications and authorizations. They will also require standard coding and classifications systems for health data and unique identifiers for all employers, providers, and health plans. Finally, HIPAA will require compliance with a set of security standards designed to ensure confidentiality when electronic data is exchanged.

Vendors should be aware of the effect these impending requirements will have on their EMR systems, and they should also have a specific plan in place for upgrading their system for HIPAA compliance. Question vendors closely regarding this issue.

Which product should you select?

The answer centers around several critical elements of design and implementation. The burden of selecting a system may seem overwhelming, but several steps can simplfy the process. These following criteria do not cover all possible functions, but they do represent those that contribute most significantly to overall success. Ask for a product demonstration in each of these areas:

1. *Timely and effective clinical decision-making support.* Physicians need immediate, easy access to information to measure or improve the quality of care. Will the product meet both the physician's need for decision support at the point of care and the organization's need, if it is part of a health care system, for access to information? Both attributes are significant.

2. *Clinical workflow automation.* EMR should emphasize all aspects of workflow affecting patient care, not just patient encounter. It must improve clinical communications between care providers. Does the system work the way physicians do? How does the EMR help the clinician know what to work on next?

   ■ The software should automate the management of encounters, clinical communication, and unsigned documents.

   ■ Will the product improve communication among clinical staff? Can care providers manage most patient issues without having to meet face-to-face?

   ■ Does the product automate the review of external reports, such as lab results and consultations? Does it file them in the correct chart and present them to the physician as unsigned documents? Does it automatically highlight abnormal lab values and display them in the context of a longitudinal flowsheet?

   ■ Will the program allow clinics to identify and reach a target population in order to meet organizational goals on the level of care provided?

   Example: If your most recent HEDIS report shows your clinic is performing below the Public Health Service goal for cholesterol screening, the program should identify those adults under your care who have not received a screening in the last five years. It can then automatically generate personalized letters advising them of this and other tests for which they are now due.

3. **Effective data entry.** The software must ensure that key problems, medications, observations, and results are well structured and consistently coded while simultaneously allowing flexibility in entry methods for unstructured notes. Data entry techniques vary widely; some users prefer cascading pick lists, which is a technique for organizing vast amounts of specific information in flowsheet or decison-tree form, while others find that text templates maximize efficiency.

Since uncoded data are almost impossible to analyze accurately, it is critical that data needed for analyses are collected in a well-structured and consistently coded format. Data must also be collected in a standardized way if it is to be pooled across patients, providers, and settings. Finally, care team members must be able to have simultaneous access to the record in order to maximize communication across the team and to enable clinicians to work in parallel. To evaluate data entry in a system, consider:

■ Does the system support a mixture of data entry techniques? Does it force you to enter data in a particular order, or does it readily enable you to respond to additional data from the patient?

■ Can mechanisms for data entry and review be modified to meet specific needs of an organization, practice setting, or specialty? Does the system adapt to the differing needs of both computer novices and a "power users"?

■ Does the product let physicians and nurses document encounters simultaneously, or does one lock the other out? Are data entered by the nurse immediately visible to the physician?

■ Does the system support the entry of structured data, using standard vocabularies, as a natural by-product of documenting the encounter?

   Example: The problem list lets you use SNOMED coding to capture problems that may influence clinical decisions without forcing you into a diagnosis. For instance, on the active problem list you can record that a patient has a family history of substance abuse and is showing symptoms of severe depression without entering a formal diagnosis of depression.

■ Does the system let you capture and track health assessment data using a formalized vocabulary? Does it use LOINC or other controlled vocabularies to ensure that results from the same tests from different labs are meaningful when compared both across patients and over time?

4. **Informed clinical review.** The program must offer quick access to pertinent information in a way that increases the confidence and quality of decision-making. If a physician can quickly comprehend a patient's history and response to care, he or she can quickly develop a better-informed treatment plan. A well-designed software program puts this kind of information in front of the clinician in the fewest number of steps, summarizing problems and linking them to actions taken. Information should be presented in a specialty- or problem-specific manner.

■ Does the product create a problem-oriented record that links actions with problems, enabling rapid focus on a specific problem and its course of treatment?

   Example: You are covering for Dr. Foster when a patient whom you have never seen before arrives with symptoms of an upper respiratory infection. You instantly organize the chart so that you can review just the occasions on which Dr. Foster has seen the patient for asthma. You can now view previous instances of upper respiratory infection, which medications have been used previously in her treatment, and how effective they have been.

- Does the product organize structured data so that you can review vital signs, examinations, lab values, and health risk assessment over time? Does it let you graph such data in a problem, panel, or specialty-specific format?

5. ***Concurrent and retrospective analysis.*** The program should support decision-making at the point of care and throughout the organization, storing clinical information so that it facilitates meaningful analysis. Decision support tools must be readily available to physicians and accessible to ensure information management and reporting. More than merely an electronic version of the paper chart, a well-structured database enables the clinician to readily determine the health status of an individual patient, a family, or the entire patient population.

The software product should also enable clinicians to perform their own queries for immediate information at the point of care and be capable of generating reports on performance and outcomes derived directly from clinical data (rather than from less accurate claims data). Population-wide analysis of clinical data is also crucial in meeting the increasing demands of payers and providers for reporting on quality and cost of care.

- Can the clinician readily determine which tests are due for a patient, based on that patient's problem list or treatment plan?

  Example: A patient with asthma calls requesting a medication refill. Before you authorize the prescription, EMR might reminds you that a year has passed since the patient was last tested for theophylline toxicity.

- Can physicians easily run their own specific queries?

- Can the software produce Health Data Information Set (HEDIS) or other performance measurement reports? For example, can the electronic medical record determine performance on measurements that depend on access to clinical data, such as quarterly HgbA1C testing for patients with diabetes mellitus?

- Can organizations write their own reports or access the database from third-party products (e.g., spreadsheets, word processors, and presentation software) for review and analysis?

  Example: Your health system is involved in an outcomes analysis study. It needs information on all patients treated with steroids over the last three years. It extracts this information from the computerized medical record and merges it into its own outcomes database using an interface utility.

Training and Support Services

Any new product that you or your health care system purchases requires integration into your current office flow and existing computer system. The integration process involves upgrading or adding new computer hardware and a network.

- *Assign a system administrator.* You must assign various responsibilities regarding the long-term upkeep and maintenance of the system. Your office manager, who will rely on expert help from outside your office, will assume many of these functions.

- *Train your staff.* Your existing staff must train to use the software and to care for and use the network. Training involves all office staff and physicians. The training support for office automation, therefore, must be coordinated accordingly. (Chapter 2 presented more information on preparing your staff through training.)

Following your initial purchase, support and maintenance can become your greatest EMR-related expense. Many medical software companies generate revenue through supporting their own products. Charges may be attached to many services. Be sure to negotiate the following support services as a part of your initial discussions with your potential vendors.

- Training materials, on-site personnel for initial training, and product updates are all obvious services that the purchaser needs.

- The vendor may charge you for consulting advice on other areas of your information systems network.

- If you have a problem that you believe is the vendor's fault, and the vendor researches it, only to find out it was the fault of another component of your system, the vendor is justified in billing you for their time.

- One way of decreasing your support costs in the future is to gain self-sufficiency for upkeep and maintenance of your system. Plan for a strategy of independence early in negotiations with vendors. Identify personnel who will be responsible for the maintenance and authorized to update your computer system, and have them available to learn from the expert. Your goal should be to get as much support service as you need to keep your staff up to speed. Your personnel will, in turn, care for your system better than an outside vendor.

Confidentiality and Security

The confidentiality and security issues are some of the most wide-reaching legal and ethical aspects of medical information. Confidentiality of the medical record is a legal privilege that belongs to the patient. Only the patient can impart this privilege to others. The physician is ethically and legally bound to protect the patient's confidentiality at all costs. Any system, electronic or not, that conveys medical information must, therefore, also protect the rights of the patient.

One benefit of automation, on the other hand, is that numbers or complexities are not daunting to the computer. Once stored, information may be manipulated at will with speed and accuracy. Many quarters of the health care industry want patient data, from the Centers for Disease Control and Prevention surveying the influenza season, to a research university deciding the relative merits of a particular cancer treatment, to a physician negotiating with a preferred provider organization. There is a legitimate need for significant information from office automation. The basic question is, Where should you store your information, and who should have access to it?

The simple answer is: *you will store your office information on a local or remote server, and as the patient's physician, you will distribute it to whomever you think might benefit from it and has a legal and ethical right to it.*

This issue raises more questions than there are currently answers. Those who believe they have a right to medical information, whether on an individual chart or aggregate information, will want to use electronic technology to access your charts. As you develop your overall information system strategy, keep these issues and the options in mind to formulate answers about rights to information.

The issues

- With whom do you have the legal right to share patient information?

- If you are an employed physician, does your parent health care system have the right to the information in your patients' charts?

- To what extent can they study this information?

- What safeguards can they build into the system to allow access only to those deemed to have proper authority to view charts?

- Does the patient have the right to restrict where his or her chart can reside?

- What security safeguards and access controls are in place to ensure that one cannot alter information in medical charts?

- Are results of medical care queries discoverable in a court of law if the user is not collating the information for the purposes of peer review?

- Can information regarding discrete populations that can be collated based on any demographic profile be sold for commercial purposes such as direct marketing?

A good software package will have several features that enhance security and confidentiality. Since all information in a medical record is sensitive, access must be limited.

- *Access hierarchy.* The software should allow different levels of access to a patient's chart according to an established hierarchy of staff members. For instance, a receptionist, whose primary job functions pertain to scheduling and maintenance of patient demographic information, should not be able to add or remove diagnoses or medications. These tasks, however, are ones your nurse might need to execute. Particularly sensitive data, such as HIV test results, can be further secured. Most software companies are particularly sensitive to security issues and have addressed these questions in their programming.

  In many ways, an electronic medical record offers more security than a paper chart. Accessing an electronic chart and obtaining information requires having a computer linked to the same network, training to use the software, knowledge of passwords and other access codes, and knowledge of how to look for a specific chart—not a likely combination of skills for a typical "hacker" to have. (People who obtain unauthorized access to computer networks, usually with sinister motives, are called "hackers.")

- *Access lockout.* Medical information should always be kept out of view of the casual observer. Just as you would not leave a patient's paper chart in the presence of someone else, do not leave an electronic chart open on a computer screen. Always "lock" the computer (using a password-protected screen saver or other safeguard software) or log out of the system when you leave the exam room. This protocol, which should involve very few keystrokes, should be the first on the list of computer habits you and your staff learn.

- *Network access (electronic "firewall").* A Wide Area Network (WAN) involves a network of LANs using high-speed communication lines (T1 and ISDN are two types). Since it is possible to have virtual, instantaneous communication between the LAN and the WAN, security becomes of even greater concern when transmitting information over a WAN. Physicians should establish appropriate safeguards before sending patient information over a network. An electronic "firewall" of security measures is one way to insure appropriate access. One possible system might involve the use of "permission codes," whereby a patient's primary care physician would electronically approve the viewing of the chart by a referral physician. Another security measure could be to have patients carry a coded or imprinted card that would enable physicians to access their charts. These cards would especially be useful if the patient shows up in the emergency room without the knowledge of the primary care physician.

- *User tracking.* A computerized system allows you to track all access to information, recording who viewed or changed any piece of data in the system. Each user leaves a *fingerprint* on his or her activities within the system. This feature becomes critical in investigating breaches of confidentiality.

- *LANs.* The most common custom for those offices that currently use EMR is to have their information reside locally on a server, with information sharing through interfaces with laboratory and billing software systems. This information sharing differs little from what happens manually today. Most LAN systems are connected to the outside world by a modem, which allows individual providers to use the system remotely. Because of these connections, LANs are not secure from determined hackers, but routine users of the system are usually in a controlled physical setting, i.e., your office, and of a known and limited number.

When you are evaluating software systems and speaking with vendors, be sure to ask pointed questions about the types and number of security features. The more safeguards that are in place, the less likely it is that unauthorized personnel will gain access to confidential patient information. Finally, be sure to stress to your staff the importance of following security protocols on a regular basis to ensure system integrity.

Practice Management Reporting

EMR reporting allows the physician and the staff to review and assess the various operational aspects of the medical practice.

At the end of a workday, you may want to know how many patients you have seen.

During the fall season of the year, your practice nurse may want to project how many influenza vaccinations he or she needs to order.

The nurse may need to know how many fiberglass casting supplies to purchase for the winter's "fall and break" season. Because these have an expiration date, buying too many wastes money.

The office manager, who uses a flexible schedule to reduce overtime, wants to know peak hours for phone calls and office visits.

The hospital administrator with whom you are negotiating a contract wants to know your economic impact on the hospital due to admissions and tests.

EMR reporting tools easily incorporate into your practice style and can have significant influence on practice efficiency and negotiating position with another party. Your electronic medical record program should be able to generate both standard and customized reports. Following are several examples.

- **Practice profiles.** One type of standard report is a simple profile that breaks down your practice into payer mix, e.g., 30 percent Medicare, 40 percent fee-for-service, 15 percent HMO, etc.

- **Practice demographics.** Another standard report is a practice demographic profile regarding age, sex, and even location based on a specific parameter, such as zip code. These elementary profiles should be quick and easy to create without additional software or "help" from the vendor.

- **User-defined reports.** Your EMR program should also have the capacity to generate user-defined reports. Customized reports are helpful, for instance, if you are negotiating with an HMO. If the HMO broaches the subject of a quality assurance program, you can quickly respond with data. As one example, you can tell your EMR to generate those charts for your patients with the diagnosis "insulin-dependent diabetes mellitus using ICD-9 code 250.01" for males whose birth date is between January 1, 1940 (01/01/40) and January 1, 1960 (01/01/60). This report will allow you to audit your documentation for middle-aged diabetics. With this feature, you can demonstrate appropriate medical care and follow-up before signing a contract.

- **Follow-up reports (letters and reminders).** The ability to generate follow-up reports is an extremely reliable function of an EMR. Your staff can use it to remind patients of follow-up visits, routine screening, or simply to see how a patient is doing with the treatment you prescribed. With a few keystrokes, staff should be able to generate a customized letter for any part of your practice.

Patient Satisfaction Benchmarking

A vast, though sometimes unrecognized, difference exists between the physician providing good medical care and the patient having a good medical care experience. Factors unrelated to the physician's actual medical decision-making often define patient satisfaction. In fact, patients who are upset with an encounter most often become distressed *before* seeing the physician. Being placed on hold without being able to state their need agitates patients. Harried employees upset patients when they give the impression they are overworked and inconvenienced. Waiting for longer than a few minutes annoys patients. Don't forget to take patient satisfaction benchmarking features of EMR into consideration when you are considering different vendors and software packages.

- Computers now can display graphical information quickly, including photographs, as previously mentioned. Being able to attach your patient's picture to the EMR record is a useful feature. Knowing the face of the patient personalizes each encounter. Being short-tempered with your patients (even over a telephone call) is less likely when you are staring at their photographs.

- The receptionist puts patients on hold less frequently with the use of the electronic medical records. Instant availability of information to your front-office staff greatly reduces the time for call transfers and scheduling.

- Your EMR system can monitor patients' waiting room times and give regular reports to your office manager for early intervention. Even in a well-managed office, physicians inevitably get behind in their schedules. If a child walks in with a laceration and requires sutures, for instance, you may fall an extra half-hour behind. Because your EMR can tell you how far behind you are, you can make small changes in procedure to improve patient service.

- Intervention can greatly alleviate your patients' frustration. Your office policy may be that if you are thirty minutes behind, the receptionist is to immediately tell all waiting patients. With this information, they can then adjust their schedules accordingly and reschedule if necessary. EMR can prompt your staff to extend this common courtesy and forestall any hard feelings. Informed patients are understanding patients.

Enhancing patient satisfaction is a common goal for every medical practice. A happy staff, good phone skills, timely appointments, and a short wait time all influence the mood of the patient before the physician ever records his or her chief medical complaint. In this respect EMR, with all its benefits, can improve the patient's attitude about his medical care, which is a genuinely positive therapeutic adjunct!

Customizing the EMR to Your Practice and Office

Your patients want to feel that you, as their physician, are in complete control of their well-being. Part of that is feeling that you recognize them as individuals. Your use of office automation should support and extend this aspect of the patient-physician relationship and reflect your personal approach to patient care. No physician wants to implement a computer system that leads to a cookie cutter method of providing health care.

- *Workflow.* A major benefit of implementing an electronic medical record system will result from your earlier examination of workflow. This exercise entailed a close look at inefficiencies, many of which can be addressed while your vendors are building and customizing your EMR system. It also revealed your unique practice style. The mark of a good EMR customization is that it will take that practice style into account and accentuate it while providing the economies and efficiencies you seek.

- *Handouts and prescriptions.* One simple way to maximize efficiencies while enhancing your practice style is using EMR for the distribution of prescriptions and patient education handouts. In such a system, the physician selects appropriate documents with a few clicks of the examining room computer mouse. After sending the documents to the printer near the front office, for a personal touch, the physician walks with the patient to the printer, signs prescriptions, and gathers handouts that have printed (all personalized with the patient's name). Pointing out any other care, such as blood draws, that they might need and bidding farewell complete the process. This gesture will benefit patients without being inefficient. Adding 15-20 seconds per patient visit can be a worthwhile investment in your patients' satisfaction, and the electronic medical record system seamlessly assists you.

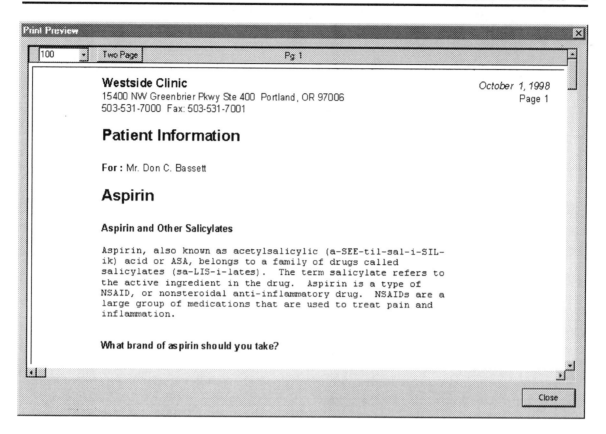

Using Purchased Databases

Computers bring a wealth of information to every patient visit in your office. A vast array of knowledge is at your fingertips; formerly, someone had to find it manually. Your information system's capacity to make these databases available enables you to greatly streamline your practice. Most medical office databases are available by subscription, with updates generally arriving at least every quarter.

- *Updating diagnosis and procedure codes.* Collection problems threaten economic existence if the physician is not familiar with proper diagnosis and procedure codes. With a paper chart system, a physician generally writes the diagnosis and someone from the front office then looks up and enters the appropriate codes. SNOMED, ICD, and CPT codes are the major code set, but there are others as well for items like "place of service." Physicians regularly attach these to patient encounters so that payers will reimburse their efforts. EMR should have all these standard codes available in an easily searched database, and the database should be updated at least once a year. EMR software available on the market today now lets the physician code the visit at the same time he or she records the diagnosis. Best of all, the entire process takes less time than it used to take to write the diagnosis down!

- *Updating patient handouts.* A useful feature to consider for your EMR system is the ability to add your own handouts to its database for easy retrieval. Commercial handout products are available for both general and specialized areas of medicine, including medication side effects, drug-drug interactions, disease conditions, presurgical instructions, and various other data you may want to retrieve. These products should also be updated annually to ensure that the most current information is available to your patients.

- *Automated updates to informed consent.* The information you can generate and give to a patient greatly reinforces the concept of informed consent. Using only a few keystrokes, for instance, you can now arm diabetics with a personalized handbook with reference information on diet, exercise, foot care, how to use their insulin, and the complications of diabetes. This information not only helps patients understand their disease but also offers documented proof that the physician has taken all appropriate steps to inform them about their disease.

Exhibit 4–4   Patient Handouts #2

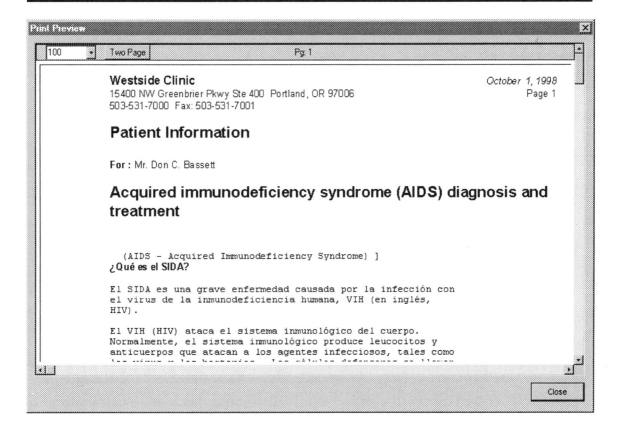

- *Decision-making software.* Practice protocols have become commonplace in medical care. These patient care pathways aid in developing standards of care. While the responsibility of decision-making still lies with the physician, you should be able to refer to practice protocols at will. Software is now available that can bring some of these decision-making capabilities to the physician's computer. The user can then easily pull "outcomes data" from these electronic pathways.

Evaluating, purchasing, and customizing your EMR may initially seem daunting. If you first examine your practice and your needs, you will enter the process two steps ahead of the game, and you will probably already have a fair idea of the kind of package you are looking for. When you evaluate vendors, you will know what to ask for and what to negotiate in terms of training and support, because you have already thoroughly analyzed your individual practice style. Finally, customizing your system will maximize the performance of your system, eventually paying you high returns on your investment. In the next chapter, we will examine ways to measure and evaluate the benefits you receive from your EMR system.

CHAPTER 5

Evaluating Return on Investment

Taking Inventory

The use of computerized patient record systems offers a variety of benefits to physician practices, as we have covered in previous chapters. For example, by providing real-time patient status reports, test results when they are available, and graphs and flowsheets of test trends, the quality of care provided can improve. Electronic medical records can help reduce costs by eliminating many manual functions and the supply and staff expenses associated with these functions. Finally, they can give practices the data necessary to attract and negotiate favorable managed care contracts.

Studies show that medical practices can realize efficiencies and cost savings by using a computerized system. In this chapter, we have identified two sources for their notable work in return on investment studies. These researchers have prepared extensively to gain the information in their reports and deserve recognition for their research. Use of their material in no way serves as an endorsement for either product or services.

In an article titled "Computerized Patient Records Benefit Physician Offices," published in the September 1997 edition of *Healthcare Financial Management*, Alan Bingham reports on the differences in efficiency between paper-based and electronic medical records systems. In the following excerpt, he reports findings related to all "file-related actions," which as a category includes documenting and filing patient encounters, test results, correspondence, phone messages, and consultations.

> *Total file-related actions occurring in one day was 360, or 45 per hour, in an optimally efficient, paper-based practice. An integrated computerized patient record system can reduce manual file-related activities dramatically and reduce or eliminate the need for a records clerk, for a typical potential savings of $26,000 per year in salary. In addition, efficiency and productivity are normally improved because charts no longer have to be moved or risk being misplaced, and because more than one person at a time can work with a chart.*

> *Based on average costs at the model clinic, which has a patient population of about 14,000 patients, the costs of a paper chart, including the folder, contents, and shelving, amounted to about $3 per patient. Paper charts, therefore, cost the clinic $42,000. In a new clinic, this cost would be saved, and in a clinic that is converting to a computerized patient record, future expenditures would be either eliminated or reduced significantly.*

> *Physicians spend four to ten hours per week on documentation, such as updating patient records, ordering tests and prescriptions, and writing progress notes, consultations, and referrals. In the clinics with fully implemented computerized patient record systems, most of these documents are generated as by-products of the patient encounter.*

Based on information from the study, clinics with computerized patient records systems in place, by the end of the first six months of system use, an 80 percent reduction in documentation time is a reasonable expectation. For a physician who spends four hours per week on paperwork, this would mean time savings of 3.2 hours per week. If the physician used this freed-up time to see thirteen more patients (at 15 minutes per patient encounter) at $55 per patient (average cost of a patient visit at the model clinic), an additional revenue gain of $715 per week would be realized. Expressed another way, $715 is the opportunity cost per physician of not implementing a computerized patient record system.[3]

Using Measurement Tools

If you would like to perform your own payback analysis, you may want to begin with the following exercise, reprinted from MedicaLogic's "Selecting an Electronic Medical Record: Measuring the Field," to discover your savings. This template is only a starting point, but you can customize it to methodically evaluate an electronic medical records purchase. It requires you to deliberately define the costs, risks, and benefits that are most applicable to you and to define the significance of each of these.

The exercise is divided into three steps:

1. Estimating your costs
2. Estimating your benefits
3. Comparing your scenarios to invest and not-to-invest

Follow these instructions as you fill in your worksheet:

1. Come to a consensus regarding the specific costs and risks associated with the investment you are considering. Some will be tangible (software, hardware, services, etc.) and others will be less tangible (resistance to change, business disruption during the transition).

2. Rank the relative importance of each decision criterion by assigning it a "weighting factor." The sum of all weights must equal 100, and the weight assigned should represent the overall cost of each factor to your organization over the period you consider to be your planning horizon. (Some costs will be one-time capital expenses, while others may be recurring.)

3. Enter the weighting for each of your identified risks or costs in the column titled Value or Weight Factor.

4. Estimate, on a scale of 0-5, the likelihood of each cost or risk manifesting if an investment is not made in electronic medical records, with 5 being "highly likely" and zero being "highly unlikely." Enter this number in the column labeled Probability Rating under the heading Without EMR. Do this for each cost item you have listed.

---

3 Reprinted, by permission, from *Healthcare Financial Management,* September 1997. Copyright 1997 by THE HEALTHCARE FINANCIAL MANAGEMENT ASSOCIATION.

5. If you are doing this evaluation through an electronic spreadsheet, you can set this "likelihood score" to be automatically multiplied by the weighting factors you already determined above, filling in the column under the heading Score.

6. If you are doing this exercise manually, multiply the two numbers and enter the product in the appropriate cell.

7. Do the same for the column that assumes you do invest in electronic medical records. Only evaluate the cost or risk associated exclusively with EMR. (For example, if you are going to upgrade your computer system whether or not you implement electronic medical records, do not associate the system expense with the medical records decision. However, if the system requirements are greater because of the electronic medical records program, use *the cost difference* between the two systems under consideration to evaluate risk associated with EMR.)

8. Add the numbers in each of the two Score columns. The totals represent the relative costs of not investing and investing, respectively.

9. Repeat the process for estimating your benefits. Use language to describe a benefit positively, such as "ability to reduce transcription costs" rather than "transcription costs."

10. When you have completed the estimates, compare your totals; the option with the highest overall score will be your best choice.

Exhibit 5-1   Investment Assessment Worksheets

Part 1: Assessing Costs and Risks						
Comparison of costs under two scenarios:		**Without EMR**			**With EMR**	
Tangible Financial Costs and Risks (50% of total weighting)	Value or Weight Factor (%)	Probability Rating (0-5)	Value x Rating = Score.	Probability Rating (0-5)	Value x Rating = Score	
Acquisition of new infrastructure required by EMR (hardware, network, etc.)						
Cost of EMR application and modules						
Cost of EMR implementation services and training						
The cost of required interfaces (development and consulting)						
Overtime pay during the first month of EMR (e.g., entering patient data, etc.) and lost physician productivity						
Cost of ongoing product upgrades and support						
Cost of future training for new employees						
Cost of ongoing network administration required by EMR application						
Total tangible costs and risks						

Exhibit 5-1 continued...

Intangible Costs and Risks (50% of total weighting)	Value or Weight Factor (%)	Probability Rating (0-5)	Value x Rating = Score	Probability Rating (0-5)	Value x Rating = Score
Provider and executive time needed to make project succeed					
Viability of vendor					
Employee and provider resistance to change					
Business disruption during transition					
Need for increased staff skills and training; higher labor costs					
Failure of product to deliver benefits promised by vendor					
Confidentiality and security of patient records					
Total intangible costs and risks					
Total Tangible and Intangible Costs and Risks					

Worksheet 2: Assessing Tangible and Intangible Benefits

Comparison of costs under two scenarios:		**Without EMR**		**With EMR**	
Tangible Financial Benefits (50% of total weighting)	Value or Weight Factor (%)	Probability Rating (0-5)	Value x Rating = Score	Probability Rating (0-5)	Value x Rating = Score
Increased revenue through improved:					
Coding accuracy					
Charge capture/billing integration					
Patient care reminders, alerts which generate preventive care					
Speed of receivables collection, and reduction in billing penalties or rejections					
Physician productivity					
Bonus from payors (incentives for quality of care, records, etc.)					
Ability to bill for home care oversight					
Costs that are reduced or avoided through:					
Labor savings in medical records, lab report filing, referral coordination, billing, reduced telephone callbacks, complying with reporting requirements (e.g., HEDIS), etc.					
Reduced copying and storage of records					
Malpractice exposure or premiums reduced					

Exhibit 5–1 continued...

	Value or Weight Factor (%)	Probability Rating (0-5)	Value x Rating = Score	Probability Rating (0-5)	Value x Rating = Score
Reduction in transcription volume					
Reduction in loss from prescribing non-formulary drugs					
Reduction in charting, other supplies					
Total tangible benefits: A comparison					
Intangible Benefits (50% of total weighting)	Value or Weight Factor (%)	Probability Rating (0-5)	Value x Rating = Score	Probability Rating (0-5)	Value x Rating = Score
Quality of patient care (20% of total weighting)					
Improved chart availability					
Greater availability of patient educational materials					
Ability to provide timely preventive care					
Ability to reduce time between patient visit and chart notes or lab results entered in medical record					
Ability to improve care from home while on call, or when covering for other providers					
Ability to improve medical records accuracy, thoroughness and consistency across the clinic or enterprise					
Improvements to the quality of Member/Patient Service through changes in: (10% of total weighting)					
Clinic staff's response time when patients call for information that requires accessing a medical record					
Turnaround time on refill requests					
The amount of time patients spend filling out paperwork					
Reminders from the clinic about preventive services					
The quality of patient education materials available					
Improved Professional satisfaction from the ability to: (5% of total weighting)					
Improve the quality of medical care providers feel able to deliver					
Improve the quality of patient service providers feel able to deliver					
Reduce the number of hours spent per week on paperwork					
Improve the ease of providing summary information to specialists					
Increase the time available to spend with patients and practice medicine					
Strategic benefits from changes in your ability to: (15% of weighting)					

Exhibit 5–1 continued...

Build market share					
Improve physician allegiance					
Win major contracts					
Increase perceived leadership in market					
More profitably assume financial risk					
Increase ability to recruit and retain physicians					
Total intangible benefits: A comparison					
Total tangible and intangible benefits					

Worksheet 3: Total Investment Assessment			
Comparison of costs under two scenarios:		**Without EMR**	**With EMR**
		Value x Rating = Score	Value x Rating = Score
Total benefits			
Minus total costs and risks			
Equals difference			

Checklist for Successful Transition

A *successful* transition from paper charts to electronic medical records is founded on these guidelines:

1. Start with a plan.

2. Set objectives.

3. Follow a disciplined evaluation process.

4. Select vendors with similar cultures and attitudes.

5. Develop a plan for your employees and your long-term staffing requirements.

6. Define the scope of the tasks to be considered and the future areas that you may include.

7. Use the "partnership" concept to create a mutually beneficial environment with your vendor.

8. Insist on service agreements; maintain a well-trained staff to keep your system up and running.

9. Develop a plan for application. Recognize that communications will be a critical success factor.

10. Plan for change.

Glossary

The following list is not all-inclusive. Knowing where to start and stop in compiling a glossary is difficult, because technology advances at such a rapid pace that a list one compiles today is often out-of-date next year (maybe sooner).

For a comprehensive resource on computer technology, you may want to visit the World Wide Web on the Internet. Many terms in the list are from the PC Webopaedia web site at http://www.pcwebopaedia.com. Others are from the National Library of Medicine, which is a part of the National Institutes of Health, at http://www.nlm.nih.gov.

Application

A program or group of programs designed for end users. Software can be divided into two general classes: systems software and applications software. Systems software consists of low-level programs that interact with the computer at a very basic level. This includes operating systems, compilers, and utilities for managing computer resources.

In contrast, applications software (also called end-user programs, e.g., EMR) includes database programs, word processors, and spreadsheets. Figuratively speaking, applications software sits on top of systems software, because it is unable to run without the operating system and system utilities.

Backup

To copy files to a second medium (a disk or tape) as a precaution in case the first medium fails. A cardinal rule in using computers is *back up your files regularly.* You can back up files using operating system commands, or you can buy a special-purpose backup utility. The term "backup" usually refers to a disk or tape that contains a copy of data.

Bits per Second (BPS)

How fast the modem can transmit and receive data; the higher the BPS, the faster the modem.

CD-ROM

Abbreviation of Compact Disc—Read-Only Memory. A type of optical disk capable of storing large amounts of data—up to 1 gigabyte, although the most common size is 650MB (megabytes). A 1-gigabyte CD-ROM has the storage capacity of 700 floppy disks, enough memory to store about 300,000 pages of text.

CD-ROMs are stamped by the vendor, and once stamped, they cannot be erased and filled with new data. To read a CD, you need a CD-ROM player. All CD-ROMs conform to a standard size and format, so you can load any type of CD-ROM into any CD-ROM player. In addition, CD-ROM players are capable of playing audio CDs, which share the same technology.

CD-ROMs are particularly well suited to information that requires large storage capacity. This includes color, large software applications, graphics, sound, and especially video.

Central Processing Unit (CPU)

The case and main data processing components of a computer, including the printed circuit boards, microchip processors, memory chips, disk drives, power source, etc.

Client-Server Architecture

Network architecture in which each computer or process on the network is either a client or a server. Servers are powerful computers or processes dedicated to managing disk drives (hard, floppy, optical, tape, etc., a.k.a. file servers), printers (print servers), or network traffic (network servers). Clients are PCs or workstations on which users run applications. Clients rely on servers for resources, such as files, devices, and even processing power.

The server is the "brain" of the office. The "client" is a workstation.

Communications Device

A machine that assists data transmission. Modems, cables, and ports are all communications devices.

Communications Software

Programs that make it possible to transmit data.

Database Management System

A collection of programs that enable you to store, modify, and extract information from a database. There are many types of DBMSs, ranging from small systems that run on personal computers to huge systems that run on mainframes. The following are examples of database applications:

- Electronic Medical Records

- Automated Teller Machines

- Flight Reservation Systems

- Computerized Parts Inventory Systems

Dial-up Access

Connecting a device to a network via a modem and a public telephone network. Dial-up access is really just like a phone connection, except that the parties at the two ends are computer devices rather than people. The capability for access to EMR away from the office is through dial-up access.

Disk Drive

A machine that reads data from and writes data onto a disk. A disk drive rotates the disk very fast and has one or more "heads" that read and write data.

There are different types of disk drives for different types of disks. For example, a hard disk drive (HDD) reads and writes hard disks, and a floppy disk drive (FDD) accesses floppy disks. A magnetic disk drive reads magnetic disks, and an optical drive (like a CD-ROM drive) reads optical disks.

Disk drives can be either internal (housed within the computer) or external (housed in a separate box that connects to the computer).

Dumb Terminal

In client-server architecture, a display monitor that has no processing capabilities. A dumb terminal is simply an output device that accepts data from the CPU. In contrast, a smart terminal is a monitor and computer that has its own processor for special features, such as bold and blinking characters. Dumb terminals are not as fast as smart terminals, nor do they support as many display features, but they are adequate for most applications.

Extranet

A collaborative network that uses Internet technology to link offices or businesses with suppliers, customers, or other businesses with common goals. The shared information can be available only to the collaborating parties or can be publicly accessible.

Fat Client

In a client/server architecture, a client that performs the bulk of the data processing operations. The actual data are stored on the server. See "Thin Client" for contrast. Although the term usually refers to software, it can also apply to a network computer that has relatively strong processing abilities.

Files

Files are all information maintained in a database about a given topic. In an electronic medical record database, all information about the practice's patients constitutes the file. All information about a specific patient forms a medical record.

Firewall

A system designed to prevent unauthorized access to or from a private network. Firewalls can be implemented in both hardware and software or in a combination of both. Firewalls are frequently used to prevent unauthorized Internet users from accessing private networks connected to the Internet, especially through intranets. All messages entering or leaving the intranet pass through the firewall, which examines each message and blocks those that do not meet the specified security criteria. See Chapter 4 for further discussion of security measures.

Infrared Transmission

A technology that allows computers to exchange data without cables, making networking within an office setting easier to achieve.

Interface

An interface is something that connects two separate entities. For example, a user interface is the part of a program that connects the computer with a human operator (user). There are also interfaces to connect programs, to connect devices, and to connect programs to devices. An interface can be a program or a device, such as an electrical connector.

Interface means to communicate. For example, two devices that can transmit data between each other are said to interface with each other.

Internet

A global network connecting millions of computers. As of 1998, the Internet has more than 100 million users worldwide, and that number is growing rapidly. More than 100 countries are linked into exchanges of data, news, and opinions.

The Internet is decentralized by design. Each Internet computer, called a host, is independent. Its operators can choose which Internet services to use and which local services to make available to the global Internet community. Remarkably, this anarchy by design works exceedingly well.

There are a variety of ways to access the Internet. Most online services offer access to some Internet services. It is also possible to gain access through a commercial Internet Service Provider (ISP).

Intranet

A network belonging to an organization, usually a corporation, accessible only by the organization's members, employees, or others with authorization. An Intranet's web sites look and act just like any other web sites, but the firewall surrounding an Intranet fends off unauthorized access.

Like the Internet itself, Intranets are used to share information. Secure Intranets are now the fastest-growing segment of the Internet because they are much less expensive to build and manage than private networks.

Leased Line

A permanent telephone connection between two devices. Leased lines provide faster data transmission and better quality connections than connection through a public telephone network, but they are also more expensive.

Local-Area Network (LANs)

A computer network that spans a relatively small area. Most LANs are confined to a single building or group of buildings. However, one LAN can be connected to other LANs over any distance via telephone lines and radio waves. A system of LANs connected in this way is called a wide-area network (WAN).

Most LANs connect workstations and personal computers. Each node (individual computer) in a LAN has its own CPU with which it executes programs, but it is also able to access data and devices anywhere on the LAN. This means that many users can share expensive devices, such as laser printers, as well as data. Users can also use the LAN to communicate with each other, by sending E-mail or engaging in chat sessions. For more information on LANs, see Chapter 3.

LOINC

An acronym for Logical Observation Identifier Names and Codes, the LOINC database is a public use set of codes and names for reporting of clinical laboratory tests and exchange of data among providers.

Modem

An acronym for *modulator-demo*dulator, a modem is a device or program that enables a computer to transmit data over telephone lines.

Network

A group of two or more computer systems linked together. (For expanded information on networks, see Chapter 3.)

PC

Abbreviation for personal computer. A single-user computer that can be used as a stand-alone system or linked together to form a local-area network. Concerning computing power, personal computers are on the low end.

Peripheral Device

Any external device attached to a computer. Examples of peripherals include printers, disk drives, display monitors, keyboards, and mice.

Printer (print server)

A printer is a peripheral device managed by the server to run print applications.

Query

Requests for information from a database are made in the form of a query, which is a stylized question. For example:

SELECT ALL WHERE NAME = "SMITH" AND AGE > 35

Report Writer Program

The information from a database can be presented in a variety of formats. Most DBMSs include a report writer program that enables you to output data in the form of a report. Many DBMSs also include a graphics component that enables you to output information in the form of graphs and charts. A good EMR will have a report writer.

Resources

Files, devices, memory, storage space, and processing power.

SNOMED

An acronym for either "Systematized Nomenclature of Medicine" or "Symmetrical Nomenclature of Medicine." It usually refers to the nomenclature and classification developed by the College of American Pathologists Committee on Nomenclature and Classification of Disease, the latest version of which is known as SNOMED International.

Storage Device

A device capable of storing data. The term usually refers to mass storage devices, such as disk and tape drives.

Tape Drive

A device, like a tape recorder, that reads data from and writes them onto a tape. The disadvantage of tape drives is that they are sequential-access devices, which means that to read any particular block of data, you need to read all the preceding blocks. This makes them much too slow for general-purpose storage operations. However, they are the least expensive media for making backups.

Thin Client

In client/server applications, a client designed to be especially small so that the bulk of the data processing occurs on the server. Although the term "thin client" usually refers to software, it is increasingly used for computers, such as network computers and Net PCs designed to serve as the clients for client/server architectures. A thin client is a network computer without a hard disk drive, whereas a fat client includes a disk drive.

Wide-Area Network (WANs)

A type of computer network in which the computers are farther apart and are connected by telephone lines. (See Chapter 3 for expanded information on networks.)

Workstation

A workstation is a type of computer used for types of applications that require a moderate amount of computing power and high-quality graphics capabilities. Most workstations have disk drives. Typically, workstations are linked together to form a local-area network, although they can also be used as standalone systems.

In networking, a workstation refers to any computer connected to a local-area network. It could be a workstation or a personal computer.

Resources

Electronic Medical Record Vendors

We do not endorse or recommend any particular product, and because the EMR landscape changes rapidly, we suggest beginning your research into vendors and products from a fresh perspective. Ask colleagues what they use. Check ads in professional publications. Run the question past your E-mail discussion groups or mailing lists.

Also, once you are ready to move forward with an EMR implementation, a fine resource to use when you are investigating EMR software is the Internet. A web site titled *Healthcare Information Systems: Web Directory of Electronic Medical Record Vendors* offers a searchable database of EMR products. The URL for this site, which does require free registration, is:

http://www.telemedical.com/Telemedical/Products/emr.html

Criteria available for the search at this site include:

- Products according to patient care settings

- Products with integrated Practice Management Software

- Products costing less than $10,000 per licensed MD

- Products with Web-based Network connectivity

- Products integrated with telemedical systems

- Products integrated with Workflow protocols

- Products integrated with Decision Support

- Vendors on the Public Stock Market

- Products that use SNOMED for data encoding

You may also wish to do preliminary research via a traditional web search, using such terms as "EMR," "Electronic Medical Records," or "Medical Records Software."

References

Bingham, Alan (1998). "Cost Justification for Computerized Patient Records." *The Journal of Medical Practice Management* 13(4):193–198.

Drill, Herb (1998). "Cyber Practice." *Modern Physician* 2(1):46–49.

Leedy, MD, Stephen A., and Rube, MD, Steven H. "The Electronic Medical Record: What and Why?" Presented to American Academy of Physical Medicine and Rehabilitation, Practice Management Seminar, Phoenix, AZ, May 1997.

MedicaLogic, Inc. (1997). *ROI: The White Paper, A Business Case for Electronic Medical Records.*

MedicaLogic, Inc. (1995). *Selecting an Electronic Medical Record: Measuring the Field.*

Nelson, Rosemarie. "Electronic Patient Records, Steps to Take Now!" Presented to Medical Group Management Association, Joint Eastern/Southern Section Conference, Orlando, FL, June 1997.

Scheese, Ronald (1998). "Data Warehousing as a Healthcare Business Solution." *Healthcare Financial Management* (February):56-59.

Index

L, M, N

O, P, Q

R, S, T

U–Z

Disclaimer

The information presented in this book is a result of the sole research, analysis, and opinion of the author.

All commercial products, publications, and services offered by persons mentioned herein are included at the sole discretion of the author.

The American Medical Association does not endorse, recommend, or guarantee, either implicitly or explicitly, any product, publication, or service offered by persons mentioned in the text or references of this book, and is not affiliated in any way with any product, publication, or person so referenced.